6 / 15 / 83

For Dr. Lewis Thomas,
Teacher of the
positive spirit.
In admiration,
Michael Fellman
+
~~Carroll~~

Anita Clair Fellman

Princeton, N.J.

Making Sense of Self_____

University of Pennsylvania Press
Philadelphia · 1981

Anita Clair Fellman
and Michael Fellman

MAKING
SENSE
OF SELF

Medical Advice Literature in
Late Nineteenth-Century America

Library of Congress Cataloging in Publication Data
Fellman, Anita Clair.
  Making sense of self.
  Bibliography: p.
  Includes index.
  1. Health education—United States—History—19th
century. 2. Social medicine—United States—History
—19th century. 3. United States—Social condi-
tions—1865-1918. 4. United States—Moral condi-
tions. I. Fellman, Michael. II. Title.
RA440.3.U5F43   613'.07'073   81-51141
ISBN 0-8122-7810-0   AACR2

Printed in the United States of America

For our parents————————————
Sara and David Fellman,
Mae Clair, and to the memory
of Harry S. Clair

Contents

Acknowledgments _____

For their readings of various drafts of our manuscript, we wish to thank John Kasson, Mary Lynn McDougall, Lewis Perry, Kathryn Kish Sklar, Ronald G. Walters, and Robert H. Wiebe. We owe a very special debt of gratitude to Donald M. Scott, who read every draft of this study with tough-minded compassion. Barbara Barnet typed and re-typed our essay with patience and good cheer. Malcolm Call and John McGuigan of the University of Pennsylvania Press made the final stages of this book preparation a great pleasure. Finally our children, Joshua and Eli, have always reminded us that there is far more to life than making sense of self.

Mt. Carmel, Haifa, Israel
May 13, 1981

Making Sense of Self

1

Making
Sense
of Self

In her lecture "Of the More Important Decisions and Essential Parts of Knowledge," which was published in 1829 in *A Course of Popular Lectures,* the reformer Frances Wright admonished her audience: "If any thing concerns us, it should be our bodies and minds. What do we understand of their structure? What of their faculties and powers? If we understand not these, how may we preserve the health of either?"[1] Forty years later, in the opening pages of the first edition of his informational medical guide *Our Home Physician,* Dr. George M. Beard, who would soon propound an influential explanation for widespread American nervousness, stressed the importance of disseminating medical and scientific information to as wide a public as possible. Only a people accustomed to looking at issues from a scientific point of view would be able to solve democratically the nation's many political and social problems.[2]

The primacy of the body and the mind, the necessity to understand and control their workings, and the application of this knowledge to the social sphere are themes which run through medical self-help guides, reform pamphlets, medical texts, and popularized scientific writings throughout the nineteenth century. Nineteenth-century Americans, of course, were scarcely the first people to be interested in these issues; curiosity about the workings of the body and the mind have characterized many peoples throughout the world, and at least as early as Aristotle, analysts have made links between the individual body and the body politic in terms of function, equilibrium between the parts, means of maintaining or achieving health and order. The anthropologist Mary Douglas generalizes that "the human body is always treated as an image of society," and she concludes that "there can be no natural way of considering the body that does not involve at the same time a social dimension." Furthermore, as Charles Rosenberg has pointed out, "It is probably fair to say that the use of disease as a sanction in enforcing behavioral norms is almost universal."[3] There have been similarities as well in much of the advice proferred by those who have sought to supply the guidance apparently needed by anxious individuals. Aristotle suggested that healthy lives were possible through the development of the human potential for moderation and balance. Probably the most popular health guide of all time, Luigi Cornaro's *Discourses on a Sober and Temperate Life,* which appeared in 1558, and has been translated and published periodically ever since, also stressed the importance of moderation in one's personal habits for health and longevity. Writing of Sir John Sinclair's bibliography to his 1807 four-volume work, *Code of Health and Longevity,* which lists 1,878 books on health and hygiene, John B. Blake concludes: "This counsel, summed up in one word, is 'moderation.' "[4]

Thus an interest approaching obsession in the self was not new to late nineteenth-century America; ideas about the origins of good and ill health had a long history, as had the advice about how to maintain or achieve good health. Virtually every debate in nineteenth-century American health guides had occurred before. Yet the collection of ideas in this body of literature, the focus, the ways in which ideas were combined, explained, and justified, had a great deal to do with a particular time and place. They do tell us much about the concerns and ideology of nineteenth-century America. Furthermore, shifting notions about the body and the mind reflected other changing social assumptions. As the social context changed, so did advice literature. Here we concentrate on advice literature that was published in the 1870–90 period.

James C. Whorton has claimed that "a thread of 'hygienic utopianism,' of belief in moral and social perfection through reform of the body, winds continuously through American culture of the last 150 years."[5] This is so only if one sees the thread as being much thicker and stronger in some decades than in others. In the 1830s and 1840s, as prefigured by Fanny Wright's always precocious reform sensibilities, the first wide-scale health-reform movement in American history blossomed. The more optimistic of reformers conjoined a glowing faith in social regeneration to belief in individual perfectionism. The first generation of popular health reformers, inheritors of both Enlightenment and evangelical legacies, asserted that the laws of nature, established by a benevolent God, would soon be discovered in toto by truly rational, faithful individuals. As a consequence, ill health and perhaps even death would be eliminated. They then proceeded to search for the key to unlock the door to the Grand Discovery—in diet, dress reform, or phrenology, to take three of their chief approaches. Faith in discoverable law, and hence in personal and social perfectibility, reached its peak in popular ideology at this time. As a result, a reformist optimism was created that characterized not only health reform, but the entire range of projects from utopian communitarianism to prison reform, from moral therapy for the mad to temperance, from feminism to radical abolitionism. Knowing and following the laws for good health would naturally lead cleansed individuals to create

5

a truly lawful and moral society which would then reproduce healthy citizens. Personal regeneration would merge into social and political perfection. The attainment of social perfectionism in the outer world would be paralleled by bodily triumph within.[6]

Starting in the 1850s, this agenda and the faith behind it began to seem less certain. The optimism of the earlier period, never shared unambivalently by all health reformers, decreased, and despair about the sources and the possibilities of the reform of human behavior increased, reaching a critical phase in the period we discuss. By the last decades of the century, faith had diminished to the more modest hope that people might be able to maintain themselves by achieving inner balance. The earlier reformers had certainly been troubled by the sickness in their society, but they thought they had a method or methods for overcoming sickness and improving their society. The shaken post–Civil War generation with which we deal decreasingly viewed the individual as a battleground of the Lord and the devil, but saw instead that same individual, buffeted by a possibly amoral nature and a potentially overwhelming social environment, nearly bereft of resources for the struggle to stay healthy and act well. Some of the earlier reformers themselves shifted ground. In 1838, Isaac Ray, a prominent founder of the Association of Medical Superintendents of American Institutes for the Insane, had based his faith in moral therapy for the insane on the premise that there was, in S. P. Fullinwider's words, "harmony between the moral and intellectual faculties" as well as between "the intellect and natural environment, [and] the moral sense and the community." By 1863, Ray feared that "artificial society, in forcing men off the land and out of stable communities, was promoting the loss of social harmony through the imbalance of mental faculties, and particularly the perversion of the 'moral sense.' "[7]

Just as institutions seemed more intractable, so, too, did flaws in the human makeup. Consequently, writers about health sometimes urged their readers to "submissively accept the results" of performing the "duties of life," and they emphasized the cultivation of "cheerfulness," surely another way of suggesting acceptance of what is, however unsatisfactory that might be.[8]

Belief in the goodness of nature and in change as construed earlier had not been dismissed or replaced, but undermined and doubted. Underlying law was far more ambiguous, and the keys to unlock the door were less shiny. The struggle, necessary as always, was more for survival and less for perfection: self-improvement was still central, but the goals were less grandiose, and the process of self-reform had become a far more difficult enterprise.

It is doubtful, as John Blake emphasizes, that the millennial aspects of the first reform movement had ever been "widely or permanently accepted."[9] Nevertheless, health reform in the 1830s and 1840s had touched a nerve, or perhaps several nerves, among a wide new American readership. The reformers' insistence that individuals were able to discern for themselves the laws of health dovetailed with an apparently widespread skepticism about formally ordained experts who appeared to use their social standing and arcane knowledge to intimidate the average person into mortgaging himself to their services. Antielitism in turn meshed with bourgeois insistence on self-control or self-repression. The self-disciplined individual was to be the basic unit through which society as a whole was to be shaped, piece by piece. The consequent development of popular self-help medicine, a trend since the Enlightenment,[10] was elaborated in America first through Thomsonian medicine, which from the turn of the nineteenth century rejected calomel and bleeding for herbs, and regularly educated physicians for the purchasable "Family Rights" to the secrets of Thomson's practice, underlined with the slogan "Every man his own physician." The success of Samuel Thomson's *New Guide to Health,* published in the 1820s by the New Hampshire farmer who became a healer, inspired the production of other American antiphysician "domestic manuals."[11] These manuals joined the earlier simplified medical practices and hygienic texts intended especially for those in the countryside who did not have access to doctors.[12] While neither homeopaths nor hydropaths, two somewhat later successful sectarian medical groups, went as far as the Thomsonians in denying the need for physicians, they, too, in their treatment and in their domestic guides appealed to the distrust of regular physicians with their crude therapeutics and elitist pretensions.

The interest in medical self-help was matched by the hunger for general information on anatomy, physiology, child care, physical education, and hygiene. The transmission of this knowledge took an even more popular form than writing—the public lecture. These lectures, which were a form of mass entertainment as well as instruction, attracted many people, including those whose religious backgrounds made them still wary of the theater.[13] The health lecture was an appropriate outing for a polite woman and eventually became an acceptable occupation for a woman. From 1838, dozens of women lecturers covered New England and the West, enrapturing thousands of their eager sisters with talks on the "Laws of Life," which might somehow provide the key not only to the family's physical well-being, but to its emotional and moral health as well.[14]

Under attack through the states' repeal of medical licensing laws, irregular medical sects, attacks on their therapeutics, the do-it-yourself aspects of domestic medical guides, and the dissemination of physiological and hygienic information by professional lecturers, regularly educated physicians began to fight back during the 1840s, partly by adopting their opponents' methods. This counterattack took many forms, especially renewed campaigns for licensing, which other writers have described.[15] Pertinent here are physicians' entry into the field of domestic medical guides, and their reworked justifications of a role as appropriate formers of the public mind. In 1854, the conservative physician William Workman spoke to the Massachusetts Medical Society, warning its members that "the 'public mind' is also reached, often misled, and sometimes corrupted, by the host of itinerant lecturers, 'professors' of 'physiology,' 'phrenology,' and 'psychology,' who gather full houses to witness their too often indecent exhibitions of manikins and pictures, and to listen to their low ribaldry and obscene jests under the guise of science." Medical men had a duty to prevent a gullible public from being duped; their "important mission" was to "instruct the people on medical subjects" in order to drive out quackery.[16]

Orthodox medical guides tended to be strictly informational texts on health and disease with a few do-it-yourself hygienic and emergency hints included; regularly educated physicians may have seen the need to provide the public with "correct" information, but they certainly had no intention of cutting off their own livelihoods. For a time, Thomsonian, homeopathic, hydropathic, and regular medical guides competed in the marketplace. By the 1870s, however, virtually all domestic medical guides had ceased giving instructions for curing cancer or setting broken bones, and instead followed in format, if not in philosophy, the educational form of orthodox guides, with the emphasis placed upon hygienic rules. The need for self-treatment diminished with increased density of settlement. The collection of large numbers of people in cities and the large-scale production made possible by industrialization also made profitable a patent medicine industry to treat those who were too skeptical, too isolated, or too poor to go to a doctor. Furthermore, with increased specificity of diseases known and with a resulting therapeutic complexity, even those belonging to irregular medical sects emphasized more and more the need for a thorough medical education for their practitioners. By the 1870s, physicians' greater capabilities to diagnose and treat their patients, as well as their concerted efforts to convince the public of their indispensability, had led to a definite diminution of antiphysician sentiment.[17]

The written advice given to people about their bodies and their minds reflects these changes in the role both of physicians and of the domestic medical guides. While the medical and scientific advice literature of the period 1870–90 includes some leftovers from the earlier period of irregular millennial optimism and orthodox medical skepticism, the literature generally played a different role in the lives of its readers than had earlier guides. However, the continued popularity of domestic medical guides, as well as the frequency with which articles concerning health appeared in middle-class magazines, indicates that the American people had by no means simply resigned responsibility for their physical and mental well-being to their physicians. While doctors were able to do more than they had been able to earlier in the century during the first health-reform movement, our study ends just when the major bacteriological discoveries would have major effects on health through the isolation of specific bacilli and inoculation against the more frightening childhood diseases, through the purification of the milk and water supplies, and through vastly refined surgical techniques and asepsis.[18] Thus the period 1870–90 portrayed in the literature is one of skepticism, with some guarded optimism at the end.

But it was not only the inability of medical science to provide a hygienic millennium which provoked the writing and the reading of the domestic medical guides, sex and marriage manuals, and popularized scientific articles which form the basis of this study; it was also the need of a changing American people to have themselves explained to themselves. In these guides, the body became the focus for a broader intellectual sorting-out. In the period 1870–90, Americans were in the midst of a process of economic and social transformation. Entering late capitalism, the trends toward industrialization and urbanization had accelerated. The American population was growing dramatically and was of increasingly heterogeneous origin. Daniel T. Rodgers characterizes America in these years as "a paradoxical society—booming, yet fragile, engaged in the march of progress yet adrift in flux, inspiring expansive hope even as it reinforced . . . fears."[19] For every one who gained through the growth and changes, there were numerous others who felt themselves outmaneuvered and shortchanged, who felt that they were not in control of their lives. Even those, who with more to invest had more to gain, were forced to endure both a society which at once sought them as new experts and resented their claims, and an uncertain economy which promoted waves of bankruptcy and panics almost as readily as it did periods of economic success. Population and productivity may have been growing by leaps and bounds, but the economy, the community, and the political arena often appeared unmanageable.

While there were hopeful moments and optimistic individuals, disorder increasingly came to appear persistent and impervious to exorcism in late nineteenth-century America. Total reform of the individual, and by extension his society, as had been an ideal in antebellum America, now seemed untenable. Yet political institutions were so corrupt that many felt compelled to form new political alliances to reclaim power on behalf of the people, and many more suffered in political silence. The modest (or immodest) goals of the small entrepreneur seemed unattainable in the presence of the monopolies that intersected with his business at unexpected points. In addition to the threats posed by weather conditions and grasshopper invasions, farmers felt themselves to be manipulated callously by the banks, railroads, and equipment companies. Wage earners' sense of self-determination decreased as their real employers became further removed from the place of employment and as their own efforts to organize were at best rebuffed by employers' and economists' insistence that to do so would be a fruitless violation of incontrovertible economic laws. Native-born Americans, aghast at urban crowding, poverty, disease, and crime, could think of no other way to explain these phenomena than to blame the nation's immigrants who, they believed, first took the jobs rightfully belonging to others and who then, by way of gratitude, applied unsuitable European philosophies and techniques of labor protest to an increasingly volatile industrial scene. The literature of industrialism focused around strikes, employed foreign workers, and outside agitators as explanations for industrial violence and expressed the middle-class authors' rage at the curtailment of self-determination in all spheres of life and their anguished desire to stretch paternalism over the gaps in indus-

11

trial relations.[20] The nativism of earlier days merged into racism as evolutionism seemed to give support to theories of racial differences, and to the greater likelihood of negative rather than positive racial qualities being transmitted from one generation to the next. Disruption entered even into the idealized middle-class household, yearned for by the aspiring as a sanctuary from the ugliness outside. Women appeared restless, viewing their sanctuary more as a prison and their masculine providers as sometime tyrants, insensitive to their needs as individuals. They spilled out of their homes into women's clubs, ready to hear from their leaders that justice demanded their self-development and that social conditions required the application of their special qualities and experience. The women's daughters were asking to be sent to universities and were informing their bewildered fathers that women, far from being eager to stay well away from the corruption outside the household, should be able to vote.[21]

While these tendencies, perceptions, and events were essential parts of the social setting against which the advice literature was written, few authors referred directly to them. To explain why all was not well, they instead focused, sometimes explicitly, sometimes symbolically, on the underlying causes of anxiety. The same economic growth that was such a source of pride was also threatening, destructive of the very community which made that growth possible.[22] One writer warned that "a moral and social gangrene pervades the community, and threatens its life."[23] He could have been referring to many disturbing changes in values that were occurring in the process of modernization, which forced changes in peoples' self-conceptions. James Gilbert and Daniel T. Rodgers have explored with subtlety the changes in American values that occurred with the transition to industrial labor, itself created by the work ethic and then responsible for rendering the old work ethic ill fitting.[24] They deal with the incongruity between the enormous increases in productivity in the United States in the last half of the nineteenth century and the compulsive anxiety to produce endlessly. The "Victorian concern with scarcity, with the economic necessity of constant doing," and the sense of "social duty to produce,"[25] expressed in William Ellery Channing's 1840 admonition that "the material world does much for the mind by its beauty and order; but it does more for our minds by the pains it inflicts; by its obstinate resistance, which nothing but patient toil can overcome" preceded the growth of the factory system at mid-century, but accompanied it as well.[26] Why should this be so? Along with the proliferation of goods produced, the changing American economy created in the years we are studying a very substantial increase in the number of white-collar workers, at a more rapid rate, in fact, than the increase in factory workers.[27] The more ambiguous relationship of these, often middle-class workers to production, may have been one reason for the persistence of the anxiety over production beyond the time when the nation's industrial output called for any self-flagellation.

Such a concern, evident in the advice literature we have studied, was intended for middle-class individuals. The transition from the more direct and modest modes of subsistence prevalent through the eighteenth century to the less direct nineteenth-century ways of producing one's livelihood, such as through working in an office as a bookkeeper, selling goods in a store, writing for a newspaper, being a corporate lawyer, banker, or stockbroker, engineer or administrator, or selling insurance, seems to have made the new white-collar workers and professionals uncomfortable at a very profound level. As S. Weir Mitchell, a Philadelphia physician who made a very comfortable living from treating diseases of the middle class, put it, with a shrewdly selective nostalgia, outdoor life, wresting subsistence from the elements, had once given participants "a sense of elastic strength." This had been the presumably less nerve-racking manner in which the ancestors of late nineteenth-century middle-class individuals had lived. "A few generations of men living in such a fashion store up a capital of vitality which accounts largely for the prodigal activity displayed by their descendents, and made possible only by the sturdy contest with Nature which their ancestors had waged." Playing upon the guilt of his only in-directly productive, but intensely consumerist, readers, Mitchell warned that they were living on their capital and were paying for it with physical and social ills.[28]

An extension of this anxiety was the argument that mental work was easier to overdo than physical labor, the signs of mental fatigue being more difficult to perceive, but, if anything, even more dangerous over a long period of time.[29] There was no comparable concern with working-class fatigue until the twentieth century. The sense of the inappropriateness and danger of the new mental pseudo-productivity in part explains the explosion of interest in sports and exercise which occurred after the Civil War, and is widely reflected in other places in the advice literature as the urgent need to rectify the imbalance between physical and mental labor.[30]

Advisors projected their anxiety over the loss of "real" productivity especially on women in two major ways. One was the scorn they heaped upon idle, fashionable, middle-class women, at the least warning them that they owed their more highly strung nervous organization to their "freedom" from manual labor, and at the extreme labeling them "beautiful tyrants, before whom everybody must make obeisance . . . just well enough to go to the opera and the play." Women exemplified all that was "rich and fashionable," that luxury which was both a desirable goal and an ensnaring lure.[31] The second degenerative manner in which women's lives demonstrated forms of productivity changing for the worse was the decreasing tendency, especially of middle-class, native-born women, to bear children. By 1880, the United States had a lower ratio of children to women of childbearing age than any country in Western Europe save barren France,[32] and the relative infecundity of well-educated white, Protestant women, in an era of intense racism, led to widespread fears of "race suicide." This perturbed many authors who were at a loss to see any compensatory new form of female productivity, and who viewed women's use of contraceptives and shameless requests for abortions as reflections of a hedonism and a decline in the values of

14

childbearing, hard work, and self-sacrifice, which they felt to be time-honored, cohesive qualities in the community.[33]

If changes in economic forms were provoking or further-ing along changes in self-conception, if, as Robert H. Wiebe argues, the traditional community could no longer provide a sufficient base for identity and comfort, and a self-confident set of professional elites failed to provide a focus for values and identity until the twentieth century, then during this time lag, the sources of identity and values were especially tentative. We be-lieve that in late nineteenth-century America a great deal of gen-eral anxiety produced by the strains of this alienating culture and everyday stress from living in difficult surroundings, and in im-personal as well as personal relationships, was focused, in a sense "introjected," into self-concern—the ways in which one's mind and body functioned, failed to function, could function better. Perceived disorder in the outer world was paralleled by an as-sumption of bodily fragility within. By emphasizing the building of personal boundaries, fears were expressed that such bounda-ries might be disintegrating, that the self was threatened within a threatened society. Not only were the mind and the body major symbolic regions and foci of general social anxieties, they seemed to offer the first and foremost potential ordering places. If in-dividuals could learn to understand and control themselves in the most immediate sense, they might gain at least the illusion of ordering their social world. People surely were eager for individ-ual blueprints with social overtones by which to delimit and evalu-ate those elements of the world which they could touch—their own physical selves for a start.

These blueprints, to us, are what constitute ideology, and we are concerned in this book with the shapes of a particular popular ideology, sought by rulers and ruled alike, and devel-oped to explain the working of the human body and mind in late nineteenth-century America. Who is it that undertook this task of teaching the public how their bodies and minds worked, and what they should do to prevent disaster and indeed to improve their performances? Increasingly the family and the churches could

15

not provide a stable and sufficient base for advice, even on these intimate questions, and ordinary men and women had to turn elsewhere for advice and comfort. In our example, they sought to comprehend their bodies and their minds by at least buying and presumably reading enormous printings of books about themselves. We have chosen to apply the terms *instructors* and *advisors* to the book authors, those secondary socializers who were called upon by late nineteenth-century Americans. They did not think of themselves, nor do we believe they were perceived as *ideologues* in the pejorative, oppressive sense with which that word is often used (although they were marshalers of ideology in the sense of the term as we have defined it). Neither do we see their advice as the artificial imposition of ruling-class rationalizations, as conscious efforts designed to frighten the ordinary citizen into docility and order.[34] The use or threatened use of coercion is not a strong but a weak exercise of power by those who shape cultures: far more efficient is moral suasion and example expressed in good (as well as in ill) faith by culture leaders to whom subjects voluntarily turn for advice. We do not mean by this definition to diminish the differentials of social power between ruled and ruler, nor to suggest some fundamental social contract or community of equals, but to expand the definitions of ideology and power as they are most often employed.

The analysis of the Italian Leninist Antonio Gramsci is especially instructive on this point. Gramsci distinguished leadership based on consent from domination based on force, the coercive state from the broadly shaped culture. "A social group can, and indeed must, already exercise leadership before winning governmental power (this is one of the principal conditions for the winning of such power); it subsequently becomes dominant when it exercises power, but even if it holds it firmly in its grasp, it must continue to lead as well."[35] In this definition of ideological hegemony, coercion is always an alternative to be used when necessary, but implied coercion does not therefore characterize every set of means of rulership. Reducing each ideological issue to an exercise of final brute power violates the range of means by which societies are ordered. This is particularly so when systematic sanctions are impossible, which is the case in most social exchanges, particularly in an individualistic, mobile society.

Leadership, after all, is widely sought by leaders and by those who are led. The entire socialization process is characterized by a real exchange between those who seek to lead, and must therefore read their subjects, and those who seek ordering principles from authoritative sources. Authority is ascribed as much as asserted. Erik H. Erikson's analysis of ego development is very helpful concerning this exchange; in fact, he merges the definition of identity-seeking with that of ideology-formulation, most precisely in the adolescent stage of identity crisis. At this stage, writes Erikson, "Each youth must forge for himself some central perspective and direction, some working unity, out of the effective remnants of his childhood and the hopes of his anticipated adulthood; he must detect some meaningful resemblance between what he has come to see in himself and what his sharpened awareness tells him others judge and expect him to be."[36]

This reciprocal, moral as well as force-centered definition of ideology is especially useful in the intensely mobile, modernizing, urbanizing world of late nineteenth-century America where a powerful industrial society was created on a premise of classlessness, without much aid from a strong or coercive state, and without the opposing thrust of a united counterculture of the oppressed. This was no homogeneous society, and, to be sure, there were openly coercive moments and institutions, but the society was held together to the degree it was by inertia, promise of rewards, and moral suasion more than by force or effective social control. Self-repression was the primary governing agency, rather than suppression from above, in a society which was liberal rather than totalitarian. This society was characterized by waste, dissent, and chaos, not by tightly dominating rulership and efficient economic and social construction. It produced not good citizens, but anxious "orphans" who were cut off from traditional ties, set adrift in new, barely comprehensible places.[37]

Consequently, we have emphasized debates as well as concordances among these late nineteenth-century instructors about the self, since they did not develop a consistent "line" which they all accepted and forced upon their audience. Instead, they discussed and argued within a range of values and possible meanings. It is this range, its inner contradictions and boundaries, and not a single coherent and clearly articulated position which might be derived from it, which constitutes the ideological blueprint within which those seeking instruction learned more about themselves.[38]

In the late nineteenth century, science had not yet been split overtly from moral instruction. Physicians and scientists, until the end of the century, employed overlapping moral and scientific categories, and they construed their task to include instruction, in the language of the day, to as wide a public as possible (best exemplified perhaps by the flourishing *Popular Science Monthly*), while they also pursued their scientific research. The two cultures, created by the drive through esoteric language and methods into deliberately detached professionalization and more covert moralism, were not nearly so divided as they are today.[39] As a check for the consistency between what physicians and physiologists wrote for the public and what they wrote for each other, we have also sampled medical textbooks and medical journals on some topics. Regular physicians and academic scientists, however, did not monopolize advice-giving about the body and the mind. Presented in general literary forms, such as nonspecialized magazines, textbooks, health and behavior guides, advice literature, taken as a whole, as a genre, constitutes the chief source for this study. We have also used material produced by clergymen who had not yet lost all traces of their former cultural leadership and by "irregular" advisors, who would not fulfill twentieth-century criteria as professionals or proto-professionals. Yet in an era of limited success in regular medical and other therapies, the line between irregular and regular blurred, especially in terms of some of the values to which they all referred and the audience to whom they projected.

Regular physicians by the 1870s were eclectics in the sense

that they were empiricists about treatments, using whatever seemed to work even without a firm theoretical base. They often approached homeopathy in moving away from the heroic dosages and purges that were common earlier in the century to more minimal therapies. Many perfectly respectable medical men used electricity and water cures and other forms of what would strike us as faddism in therapy as well.[40]

Clearly, many patients would seek treatment from both regular and irregular physicians, and the public bought books from both regulars and irregulars since they were probably more concerned with feeling better than with whatever professional divisions concern modern historians of medicine or were of significance to the physicians of the period. To a real extent, then, we feel we also should look for an ideology expressed by a broad sample of those to whom the public turned for advice. Advisors form a "group" with shared values, which is more useful heuristically than would be more careful divisions between regulars, irregulars, and nonmedical teachers. When we think it important, we point out distinctions between types of advisors. However, we are after the range, boundaries, and conflicts within an ideology offered to the public concerning the proper functioning of the body and the mind.

Our purpose here is to discuss what the instructors said, and only in a limited manner to deal with how that advice was accepted, acted upon, or rejected, which forms a rather different set of problems. However, it does not follow that instructors about the body and the mind created and imposed an ideology; rather they responded to widespread social needs, which they were only too glad to fill, for purposes of enhanced self-definition, increased social legitimacy, and financial gain, as well as for overt, instructional purposes. The need to assert their right to leadership, rather than to assume it, is indicated by the many justifications offered by the authors in the advice literature. A fine illustration is provided by Dr. Hugh Hodge's published lecture to medical students on criminal abortion in which he first states that "the duty of every professional man [is] to exert all possible influences to protect the health and welfare of individuals," and then, tellingly, he returns to this theme, saying that "it seems hardly necessary to repeat that physicians, medical men, must be regarded as the guardians of the rights of infants. They alone can rectify public opinion; they alone can present the subject in such a manner in which legislators can exercise their powers aright in the preparation of suitable laws; that moralists and theologians can be furnished with facts to enforce the truth on this subject upon the moral sense of the community."[41] Both newer and older advisors, often in loose alliance, struggled for leadership. Many Protestant clergymen, as Ann Douglas has demonstrated, searched, alongside the Dr. Hodges, for renewed constituencies amenable to their desires for leadership.[42] Thus, the advisors, themselves, were in many respects marginal men and women, with their own role anxieties as well as those anxieties they shared with other members of their culture. It is in these ways that more general social inferences might be drawn from this limited body of material. Even the most regular and conventional of physicians, for instance, were members of an anxious and fragmented profession, as Barbara Rosenkrantz has emphasized:

> At the beginning of the last quarter of the nineteenth century those Americans who assumed the calling of physician were more distinguished by competing roles and practices than by common professional standards. Definitions of disease, therapeutic procedures, and preventive hygiene reflected widely diverse training, access to institutions for the treatment of diseases, and relationships between physician and patient. Even among those physicians whose education, formal affiliation, or locus of practice prompted some common professional behavior, models of preparation and practice remained at issue at the end of the nineteenth century . . . and the absence of an effective organization on a national scale was but one reflection of the heterogeneous origins of professional expertise and authority for the care of the sick.[43]

The anxieties of physicians and other advisors came through clearly in their assertions. They published in large part to reassure others and themselves; they constantly referred to laws in nature which they could not easily find replicated in the human world: all their calls echoed their fears of lawlessness, of uncertainty, of a chaos beneath. Almost all of them shared a hope for the potentiality of the autonomous yet freely self-disciplined individual achieving equilibrium through moderation, or somehow transcending limits, and they also feared that such an individual would never be created. Similarly, the American society they saw and grappled with was both a place always tending to loss of control, and one in which law somehow still could come to function freely.

To some degree, a faith in the scientific method was emerging, but it really only mushroomed in the sector of ideology we are discussing in the late 1890s. Like the antebellum belief in total reform, the early twentieth-century belief in the scientific method was a powerful reformist faith leading to a variety of earnest projects. That faith and its projects are now in a period of decline. Skepticism and despair about the origins and possibilities of changes within individuals and in American society in general are clearly widely shared attitudes. Of course, countercurrents and lags as well as simple indifference characterize each of these periods, and we do not mean to place undue emphasis on this crude chronology, but the late nineteenth century does strike us as a period during which many basic ideological questions appeared more confused than certain. In a period of ideological doubt, such as this, the gaps within the prevailing viewpoint were more evident than they had been immediately before or after, thus allowing us more than brief glimpses at all that anxious terrain underlying self and society which neither could be avoided nor, finally, explained.

21

2

The
Healthy
Self

"The true physician supplies conditions," stated Russell T. Trall, a water-cure specialist who was strongly influenced by homeopathy, and "Nature cures." As did many health advisors, Trall then outlined his series of laws to be followed, which included:

The Hygienic System
Principles of Hygienic Medication

The Hygienic System, or the treatment of disease by Hygienic agencies, is based on the following propositions:

1. All healing or remedial power is inherent in the living system. The "properties" of drug-medicines, as they are called, are simply morbific effects.

2. There is no curative "virtue" in medicines, nor in anything outside of the vital organism.

3. Nature has not provided remedies for disease. She has only provided consequences or penalties for taking or doing those things which occasion disease, the disease itself being an effort to remove those causes.

4. Health is found only in obedience to the laws of the vital organism. Disease is the result of disobedience.

5. Health is normal vital action in relation to things usable. Disease is abnormal vital action, or action in relation to things non-usable.

6. There is no "law of cure" in the universe; the condition of cure is, obedience to physiological law.

7. There is one universal rule applicable to the treatment of all disease by Hygienic remedies, and that, to balance functional action. If this is done, no disease, however violent, will prove fatal.

9. Disease is not, as is commonly supposed, an enemy at war with the vital powers, but a remedial effort—a process of purification and reparation. It is not a THING to be destroyed, but an ACTION to be REGULATED and DIRECTED. . . .

11. Truly remedial agents are materials and influences which have NORMAL relations to the vital organs, and not drugs, or poisons, whose relations are ABNORMAL and ANTI-VITAL.

17. . . . Diseases are caused by obstructions, the obstructing materials being poisons or impurities of some kind.

18. The Hygienic system removes these obstructions, and leaves the body sound.[1]

Trall, although a regularly educated physician, practiced as an irregular physician, critical of the therapeutics of mid nineteenth-century orthodox medicine. In 1843, he opened in New York City one of the first two American water-cure establishments, and later became editor of the *Water-Cure Journal* and author of many self-help domestic medical guides. While more prone to codification of universal truths than was fashionable by the last third of the century, nonetheless, he shared with many of his contemporaries the assumption that good health was not a matter of blind good luck. As in Trall's Hygienic System, the explicit assertion of most writers about health was that nature was lawful rather than chaotic. She provided a comprehensible set of instructions for the naturally rational, average individual to follow. Obeying natural law would at least keep disease and disorder at bay. "These rules or laws for a right mode of living formulated, or reduced to a plain code, and man made aware of their importance," a typical instructor admonished, "disease should be regarded as nothing more or less than the punishment for his ignorance and the lawlessness of his behavior. There appears to be no sufficient cause why he may not become the most healthy, instead of the most sickly of beings."[2] Ideally, there was little that was arcane or difficult about the process of individual discovery of natural order. One popular health book writer thought, for example, that eating a huge evening meal was obviously "contrary to physiological law, to nature and to commonsense."[3] The ordinary person had sufficient if undeveloped internal means to choose freely to follow laws which were rooted in nature.

For their part, many advisors, physicians and nonphysicians, assumed their task to be to set their readers as directly as possible within the context of the laws of nature. The limited capabilities of physicians and the assumption that scientific laws were comprehensible and communicable to all fostered the emphasis on individual responsibility for adopting a physiologically lawful way of life. Not all health reformers had the same ends in mind, however, as they exhorted their readers to preserve their health by the appropriate means. The veterans from the earlier, perfectionist age looked forward, as Ronald Numbers puts it, "to the virtual eradication of disease in a millennium of perfect health." Others, like the Seventh Day Adventists, became preoccupied with health and healing, largely because they saw illness as expressive of the dreariness of life on earth and obedience to the laws of health as a precondition for their entry into heaven.[4] Still others had less grandiose hopes and fears, and they seemed to have felt that lawful behavior in one sphere would lead to lawfulness in all aspects of life. If ignorance of law led to immorality, then it was clear to would-be advisors that it was their duty to keep their readers informed and hence healthy and moral.

On first glance, then, this natural order was beneficent, but there were also elements of fear in it. If obedience would surely bring good health, disobedience would certainly bring down wrath in the form of bad health, and frustrated advisors were aware that humans were stubbornly prone to disobedience. "Nature is very kind when she has a chance, though she is dreadfully cruel when abused," one writer on mental health warned. Nature was both a rewarding and a punishing feminine deity, whose dictates were absolute. Moral and physical adjustment to natural order were one and the same thing, since "the human organism was a thing both material and divine."[5] Law prescribed appropriate behavior and would supply final judgment.

If nature was absolute, however, she was not capricious: the whole pattern of moral and physical behavior, not momentary acceptance or transgression of her law, would lead to her judgment. General choice of life pattern, not slips or random grace, should lead to the grant of good health. Put another way, guilt was generalized throughout life rather than specified in any single action, and willed self-control could stave off negative judgment.

> Every disease is a protest of Nature against an active or passive violation of her laws. But that protest rarely follows upon a first transgression, never upon trifles; and life-long sufferings—the effects of an incurable injury excepted—generally imply that the sufferer's mode of life is habitually unnatural in more than one respect. For there is such a thing as vicarious atonement in pathology: a strict observance of any one of the . . . principal health laws

rarely fails to reward itself by a long immunity from the consequences of otherwise evil habits.[6]

If ideally nature was the sure guide (the fears she induced notwithstanding), modern civilization in this argument was the antithesis of nature. Disease was man's product; nature was health. If man were "ever made free from [disease]," it would only be by correcting his own conduct and bringing it into "harmony with nature."[7] Both the compulsions of modern social forms and personal defections from the natural state had led men and women from right living to an intemperate, artificial effeteness.

Like the Europeans, late nineteenth-century Americans had a recurrent hunger for the primitive, a yearning to throw off the artificialities of a corrupt civilization and to return to a state of harmony with nature. It is likely that this nostalgia for a presumed earlier golden age signaled different sorts of distress with the current state of affairs depending upon when and where the romanticism was found. As regards this body of advice literature, it is likely that it reflects much rural, preindustrial nostalgia, as well as a sense of estrangement which often accompanied the late nineteenth-century transformation of social forms: rural to urban, homogeneous to heterogeneous, active producer to passive wage-earning consumer. Thus the lexicon of instruction was based on the often unconscious but prevalent assumption that in order to regain health, people would have to decivilize—to replace complex and decadent habits with behavior that was somehow simpler and cleaner. The tool for achieving this alignment with nature, paradoxically, was, for most of the advisors, human reason. Through reason, or, more specifically for some, through science, nature would be revealed and humans could learn the rules for right living which civilization had obscured. "By the powers which intelligence confers," Thomas Huxley and W. J. Youmans enthused in their textbook *Elements of Physiology and Hygiene*, "man may in great measure control the causes of disturbed health."[8]

"Nature" and "civilization" were not always self-evident categories, however, and this confusion was evident in the advice literature. How did one know what was natural or what was reasonable? Perhaps instincts were no longer a reliable guide, contorted as they were by modern civilization. And yet, had not civilization arisen because human capabilities pushed the species beyond the simple urge for self-preservation? Obviously, there had been both losses and gains in the development: "[Modern life has] the natural tendency to weaken while it refines."[9] What then was the appropriate role for instinct, and were there not instincts for evil as well as for good, or was that a contradiction in terms? One writer puzzled over the distinction between instinct and perversion: "Instinct has always opposed the abuse of drugs [and] fashion. Instinct has never ceased to urge reforms. . . . On the other hand it must be admitted that perverted appetites can become as irresistible as the most urgent natural instincts."[10]

If perverted appetites were as compelling as the most urgent natural instincts, it would certainly be difficult for late nineteenth-century Americans to tell them apart, much less disavow the perversions. Sometimes that which the conventional would ascribe to perverted appetites obviously contained elements of beauty and repose that might well be attributed to beneficent nature. H. H. Kane, a journalistic voyeur into the late nineteenth-century world of drug addiction, described his visit to an opulent hashish house in New York City in 1883 where the beauty and symmetry of his surroundings so overwhelmed him that he fled their lure in a near panic of desire, uttering feebly that the dirt, noise, and drizzle of the city streets greeting him upon his reentry into the outer world were sweeter to his ears than the "cradle of dreams" he had just left.[11] What were to be his readers' guides by which to make their choices? Neither world he described was without its dangers and drawbacks. The apparently perverted hashish house offered a realm of peace, tranquillity, and joy that must have characterized the presumed earlier golden age. And yet, if followed, this life ultimately offered shame, degradation, anguish, and pain. Kane also alluded to the unharmonious, unaesthetic, tension-producing life in the streets of New York City. Yet these negative urban characteristics were part of a larger struggle for knowledge which could eventually make life healthier, if not as simple as humankind's earlier existence had been.

Advisors, then, perceived the source of social and personal disorder and possible order in the interplay between nature and civilization. Neither pure nature nor pure civilization was attainable, and all possible combinations of the two were similarly ambiguous. What should be the basis on which individuals should pattern their behavior? Was it to be nature: just, ordered, discernible? Or was it a hard-won civilization which subdued the animalism which was pervasive in nature but no longer suitable for humans who had evolved to a supranatural, rational status above natural categories? Might not nature be evil and disordered as easily as harmonious and law-giving? Might not civilization be corrupting, destructive of health and morals, as well as elevating and progressive? Whatever source of behavior the instructors posited, they betrayed anxiety about the real possibilities of order in that source. A fundamental sense of doom always remained as the opposite side of their frequently strident hopes. Although they were advisors and would-be social leaders, these writers shared, absorbed, and reflected the fright and quest for values from those below whom they sought to instruct. Torn with ambivalence, this was no self-assured set of oppressors.

These choices were made more befuddling by the difficulties of discerning what was natural as opposed to the product of civilization. The easiest way out of this was to focus on practices that were blatantly the product of inexcusable civilized excesses. Advisors could be most strident about abuses which they could blame on false civilization: the attack on bad habits provided the most obvious means to criticism and reform. Whether or not they begged the big question about the sources of behavior, advisors tended to urge self-reform of this or that aberration, thus giving their readers the feeling that improvement was theirs for the effort. For example, in a society in which heavy eating gave visible proof of affluence and dyspepsia was generally acknowledged to be the national disease, it was natural that health writers placed emphasis on the over-civilized stomach as a leading source of abuse. In *Our Digestion; or My Jolly Friend's Secret*, Dio Lewis, a leftover transcendentalist whose route to the Oversoul was exercise, advised that the care of the stomach was the true basis of good health. "The Stomach is the reservoir from which every part of the body receives its supplies, and most of its diseases." According to Lewis, good health and longevity were due to temperate, even abstemious eating habits. Such righteous asceticism, he advocated, could lead one even to "enjoy the self-denial, and [to] pity those who are stuffing and killing themselves."[12] "Only natural appetites have natural limits," another physical educationist exhorted. The appetite for rich foods induced a disgusting gluttony. "The beer-drinker swills till he runs over, and the glutton stuffs himself till the oppression of his diet threatens him with suffocation."[13]

Disgust with overconsumption, and insistence on its correction, sometimes led to self-mortification, to an anticonsumption, antimaterialist materialism (that is, you are what you eat). Vegetarians, for instance, according to James C. Whorton, reasoned that "if immoral, un-Christian behavior were the product of depraved, uncontrollable appetites, then any stimulus to these appetites should be removed." Vegetarians felt that this "cool" and "balanced" vegetable diet had "a tendency to temper the passions."[14] Such asceticism did not seem sensible to others who were as anxious about malnutrition as about gluttony. Dr. George Beard, in general, a debunker of the warnings issued to anxious readers, downplayed the dangers of overeating and denounced vegetarians as deluded. He maintained that the food of all classes should be generous in quantity, quality, and variety and that individual experience was the best guide for the appetite. Yet the distinction needed to be made between a "truly aesthetic epicure and a common gross feeder."[15]

Not merely eating, but all aspects of daily life presented

grounds for the distortions of natural ways. If some advisors focused on one abuse, more looked for patterns of unhealthy life-styles. Modern lighting and the heady night life of the cities induced violations of the natural rhythms of work and sleep that were established by traditional rural life. Nature dictated "two symmetrical periods of vital activity and vital repair . . . and that the requisite period of rest should invariably occur at the time indicated by nature . . . the hours of darkness and comparative cold."[16] That perceived as urban artificiality, which encompassed the ambivalence about the transformation of "real" labor into "pseudo" labor, particularly affected the new middle-class woman. A feminist social critic who saw women's unhealthiness as a cultural rather than a biological phenomenon, catalogued such modern traps for women as unnourishing foods, late-night parties, lack of outdoor play for girls, and tight corseting. The artificial flowers of such a clime could never unfold into healthy, vigorous blooms.[17] For the modern businessman, an overly ambitious or unethical involvement in commerce could lead to the bankruptcy of the nervous system. Ethical behavior in business and a healthy mind and body would go hand in hand. The answer to the rhetorical question "How is the merchant to avoid that mental overstrain which comes from great competition in business?" was: "By organizing his business on a basis that will enable him to stand all honest competition without serious injury." Martin Luther Holbrook, the author of this guideline, also proferred more aid in the form of 120 pages of testimonials by distinguished men and women concerning their own good habits of moderation and regulation—but not asceticism.[18]

The conundrum was that those who were ensnared by the more fraudulent of civilization's lures were in the poorest position to free themselves by a right reading of the rules. And yet, according to many advisors, if people would remove themselves from those corrosive elements of civilization which blunted their abilities to read nature's laws, then the natural rhythms of their bodies could be restored. Inactivity, stasis, was anathema to late American Victorians who wished to believe that in all spheres, correctly informed human action would overcome its opposite, which was defined as decay rather than as repose. For them the clear lesson of nature was that balanced motion among all the equilibrated systems characterized good health. The homeopaths, among the most optimistic about the order in nature, explained the minute or "atomic" therapeutic doses they prescribed as an aid to the restoration of that equilibrium of the nerve centers which was perfect health. Their doses were intended simply to aid the natural process of reaction and resistance, for as Edward Bayard pointed out, "Nature always seeks to restore the equilibrium of her forces."[19] Ed. James, the physical culturist, offered a tersely worded regimen based on principles of circulation and balance: "The secret of health, which is the equitable, complete circulation of the fluids, may be summed up in these few words: moderation in eating and drinking; short hours of labor and study; regularity in exercise; recreation and rest; cleanliness; equanimity of temper, and equality of temperature."[20] Equilibrium was thus a behavioral as well as a physiological key; it could also be an aesthetic principle. Pictures of those stout and sound, if unexciting, late nineteenth-century presidents are conjured up by W. W. Hall's description of the ideal body: "There is a medium between being fat as a butter-ball and as thin and juiceless as a fence-rail. For mere looks a moderate rotundity is most desirable, to have enough of flesh to cover all angularities."[21]

Threatened as they were by a subversive civilization, humans could not blithely assume that nature would provide unaided for their equilibrated well-being. In every day and in every way they had to make an effort to sustain the resilience of their bodies. This was to be accomplished in part through the reform of specific habits, aimed at maintaining general body flows and balances. Although some health writers stressed one or another habit, even to the point of creating a panacea, many shared the assumption that revitalized daily habits would lead to a recapturing of natural balances and thus health. Four frequently mentioned keys were diet, rest, cleanliness, and regularly evacuated bowels. For example, one writer insisted that both physical and mental deficiencies and strengths would result from specific diets: "Persons fed too much upon carbonates may be warm and fat, but will lack muscle and nerve; those fed too much upon nitrates will possess great muscles, but will lack fat and nerve; those fed too much upon phosphates will have wide-awake brains, but will lack muscle and fat."[22] To cure insomniacs and victims of mental breakdown, another advisor insisted that in order to restore normal patterns a temporary overabundance of sleep would be necessary to compensate for that which had been lost. Cleanliness, in the sense of keeping the body purged of blockages through proper diet and exercise, was a frequent admonition. A common extension of this approach at a time when bloodletting was no longer fashionable, was the insistence that the bowels move with regularity. "Order is heaven's first law. Regularity is nature's first universal rule. . . . So it is with the desire to stool," was one such formulation, while another, intended for adolescent girls ran, "The rectum should always be empty, except for a few moments preceding its evacuation, which should occur once every day, and always at the same hour."[23]

This concern with the bowels, besides reflecting eating habits and sanitary facilities, perhaps expressed fears that the disorder which people saw around them was very deep seated, possibly embedded in the very center of the individual and his society. Similarly, the insistence upon finding and adhering to the natural body rhythms and patterns of behavior suggests fear that in actuality chaos was dominant. The inability to control, to determine, and to predict lay at the root of anxiety, personal and social. When so little else seemed amenable to control, it was crucial that human beings at least be able to regulate their own body functions.

Such habits would not suffice unless the body had the cooperation of the mind. Using terms such as *self-control* and *cheerfulness*, advisors described the links between a positive mental outlook and a healthy body. The two contrasting states of cheerfulness and depression would result inevitably in the physiological states of health and decay. "Cheerfulness, as the pervading state of mind, should be assiduously cultivated and maintained as one essential condition to bodily health. A mind continually depressed, sooner or later induces bodily ailments." One wonders what life must have been like for those individuals who had to "assiduously" cultivate cheerfulness. Self-control meant guarding against "cherishing depressing feelings," and even the most frightening occurrences in life were to be faced with a "calm courage" which would provide mental equilibrium —that "literal 'life-preserver.' "[24] Once again, the preoccupation with real work became central to the advisors' analysis of well-being. Regular, sensible work, which was the means of healthfully activating all parts of the body and the mind, would maintain self-control. Hypochondria and morbid imaginings were the products of sloth. "Many an imaginative woman who has not found work strenuous and absorbing enough to take her mind off herself, is to-day a half invalid," *Godey's Lady's Book* warned its readers, "when some stern necessity for work would have made her a healthy and happy woman."[25]

In this context of mental self-control, the very widespread interest in spiritualism and mind cure in late nineteenth-century America is not difficult to understand. Mind cure was an acknowledgement that the link between individual and social perfection was, if not broken, at least decidedly weakened. Exhortation to cheerfulness in the face of whatever was destructive to that state did not encourage examination or elimination of the negative factors outside one's own self. When self-control and positive thinking were seen in much popular advice literature as central to good health, it was a long but conceivable step to the belief that the truly spiritual mind would banish disease—and possibly even death. "It is the patient who experiences a change of thought, a conversion, that prompts him to avail himself of the healing power, by letting Spirit, which is health, have its way through him," wrote L. M. Marston, the Christian Scientist physician-president of the Boston College of Metaphysical Science in 1887. "The change takes place in him, and nowhere else

. . . all the healer can do is to help the patient to change his thought; the true healing act is between the power that heals and the person healed."[26] This argument, the most transcendental assertion of the ideal of self-control in late nineteenth-century America, was in its way the logical extension of antebellum perfectionist thinking; finding the correct key would banish disease. However, antebellum health reform had been linked to reform of the social order: sick people could not hope to form a healthy community; renewed individuals would take the proper actions to rid society of its ills. In Christian Science, a late nineteenth-century creation, and in the flourishing faith-healing sects in general, the self would be attuned to the Godhead, neatly bypassing all intermediary social levels. Disorder would become meaningless when the enlightened individual learned to float above it.

The emphases on good habits and on the powers of the mind were based on the tenacious theory that disease, whether conceived of as an invasion by outside forces or as an internal breakdown of the body, could best be avoided by a marshaling of the general and natural forces for health within the body. The increasing emphasis on the specificity of disease was counterbalanced by the prevailing theory of general body states, which in the most reductionist form produced those famous nineteenth-century tonics and panaceas which, their promoters promised their eager buyers, would cure them of everything from insanity to cancer, all out of a single bottle.[27] Even the new, late nineteenth-century science of bacteriology, which made an immediate and powerful impact on popular thought, was often subsumed in the theory of general body states. The frightful microbes were resisted by some bodies while others capitulated to them, which indicated that it was the condition of the recipient rather than the power of the invader alone that would determine the final outcome.

Therefore, hygiene—the science of the preservation of health—an earlier nineteenth-century emphasis, retained a key role in the late nineteenth-century ideology we have been discussing. Born in distrust of heroic drug cures and ineffective regular physicians, as well as from Jacksonian aversion to professional elites and esoteric knowledge, and nurtured by the belief that environment helped form character, American concern about hygiene led not only to clean air and water campaigns, but also to heretical medical substitutes such as homeopathy, herbal medicine, water cures, and even to the notion that preventive medicine would make therapeutic medicine redundant.[28] By the 1870s, a well-respected regular physician could comment that "the study of the laws of hygiene is assuming in our time, in the estimation of the public and of the profession themselves, an importance which places it above even the proper business of the profession—that of the science of therapeutics. Drugs, whether remedial or prophylactic, are falling more and more into disrepute; and it is felt that prophylactic action is infinitely better than prophylactic draughts." In their textbook, Huxley and Youmans divided the world between the enlightened and the ignorant, with the former being those who had a "steadily diminishing confidence in medication and an increasing reliance upon the sanitary influence of Nature," and the latter being those who looked instead to pills and potions.[29] By the end of the century, preventive medicine, at a time when medical interventionism at last seemed justified, far from being merely a defense against unreliable therapeutics, gave hope to William Welch, the founding father of the Johns Hopkins University Medical School, that "a large proportion of the causes of sickness and death [were] removable."[30]

Such prevention was especially important in the emerging urban conglomerates, where not merely crowding and poor sanitation, but also the ingathering of presumably weak and diseased foreign stock bred fearsome epidemics and social disruption. Perhaps the improvement of bodily health through hygienic measures would lead to the improvement of social health as well. The medical educator William G. Thompson wrote of the renewed public interest in medicine as part of "an earnest desire to learn to alleviate the growing evils of heredity and environment, especially in the overcrowded cities." He observed that "the importance of a universal knowledge of, and attention to, the laws of physiology and hygiene is becoming more and more appreciated."[31]

(J. R. Black), The Ten Laws of Health[32]

   I. Breathing a pure air.

  II. Adequate and wholesome food and drink.

 III. Adequate out-door exercise.

 IV. Adequate and unconstraining covering
     for the body.

  V. The exercise of the sexual function only for, and
     no interferences with, the
     natural course of reproduction.

 VI. A Habitation in the climate for which
     the constitution of the body is adapted.

VII. Pursuits which do not cramp or overstrain
     any part of the body, or subject it
     to irritating and poisonous substances.

VIII. Personal cleanliness.

 IX. Tranquil state of the mind, and
     adequate rest and sleep.

  X. No intermarriage of blood relations.

Hygienic writing, indeed all advisory health writing, was thus based on the premise that the sway of beneficent law which hopefully existed in nature could somehow be reestablished in the lives of each individual. Of course, such writing, which was intended to accentuate constructive possibilities, had to insist that the rudimentary nature of the body was finally sound. But men and women did not live in nature, and natural living aided by reason could at best only approximate a recovery of an asserted (and doubted) primal state of perfection. Society ominously threatened to overwhelm even the apparently most healthy individual, to say nothing of disease, that still very mysterious and powerful force which was the antithesis to the optimism of believers in good and retrievable natural law.

The source of evil and hence that of good was uncertain. Guides for the potential self thus did tend to a rigid insistence on regularity. This regularity was less a Protestant-capitalist code word for repression and denial than a compensation for anxieties over potential chaos. The insistence on rigid behavioral boundaries and natural law was the attempt to reach norms rather than the implementation of truths. The sway of law was nowhere in place, the human potential for wildness and lawlessness was not even clearly defined. Thus the insistence on conformity to a code of law was quite brittle. The assertion of health as the triumph over disease was so terribly earnest because it was so uncertain, and because disease as well as social chaos loomed so powerfully and yet undefined.

3

The
Unhealthy
Self

J ust as a potentially lawless society would presumably reduce humankind to the chaos of anarchy, disregard of the laws governing the human body would lead individuals to a breakdown of body and mind: "It is interference with nature which kills multitudes of those who die of disease, as it is the defiance of her laws which made those multitudes sick."[1] A harsh but just balance characterized such definitions of disease: health was a reward and sickness was a punishment. "Sickness is discord as health is concord," one instructor advised his readers. "If we abuse or misuse any instrument, we impair its ability to produce a perfect harmony. A suffering body is simply the penalty of violated law."[2]

Of course, one logical extension of this argument would be an insistence that humans were naturally unruly and, therefore, would bring suffering down on their own heads almost as a matter of perverse choice. But as we have discussed in chapter 2, health writers, seeking constructive suggestions for their readers, at least hoped that humans could both discover and obey natural law if they so willed. First, people had to be convinced that immutable law rather than an unpredictable Providence applied to the workings of their bodies and to the determination of health or disease. As one doctor admonished his fellows in the American Public Health Association in their 1873 meeting, "There is no class of natural phenomena which the men of all times have been disposed to look upon as being more completely exempt from the dominion of law than those which concern sickness and health. The illness of an individual appears always to have been esteemed an event entirely fortuitous, which no human prescience could anticipate and no human precaution could avert." Sickness, therefore, was frequently regarded as "an evidence of Divine displeasure," when, in truth, "the laws of health and disease in living organisms are as fixed and invariable as, in abstract science, are those of mathematics. . . . In the human race, life is often shortened by ignorant or willful disregard of the conditions necessary to the preservation of health."[3] Such an argument reinforced medical and public health practitioners' sense of themselves as pioneers, bringing light where once there had been darkness, and action where once fatalism had dominated. The plea to the general public by one popular health writer stressed lawfulness in all spheres of human activity. He argued that man's successes in the physical as well as the social and religious spheres "have one and all been gained through a knowledge of law and by conformity to it." By lawful behavior on earth, "man is but placing himself in harmony with nature."[4] This repeated use of the word *harmony* has a wistful, yearning quality.

Even though, in this part of the argument, nature was presumed good, peoples' alignment with that good, which would grant them health, was always in doubt, as evidenced by all the sickness and physical suffering which characterized that age. Thus, although the face of optimism was shone upon the advisee, it was a Janus-face for someone who lost good health and thus in his pain must have been reflecting punishment for a disobedience which he might not know or understand. The only alternative to self-doubt was to question the basic assumption about the law of nature: perhaps it was not simple and good at all. How could one know of one's lawfulness or unlawfulness? How could one bring one's behavior up to a justice that might finally be unfathomable? Such fears of justice could not be brushed aside, or finally answered, but the usual response of instructors to their concerned readership was commonsensical: immoderation of behavior was the key to ill health, and a regularity of behavior would be rewarded. Moderation was the crucial ideological basis of a good life; immoderation was seen frequently as a prime indicator of the onset of disease. Moderation was sometimes seen as the law of nature, and sometimes as the creation of civilization. At times, the same advisor would use both as the source of proper behavior.

Immoderation took two forms: excess of a mental or emotional sort—defined in late nineteenth-century language as overindulgence of the passions—and physical overconsumption, exemplified by gluttony, overwork, excessive venality. Disease in this reasoning would follow inevitably from an individual's excesses. Advisors made explicit for their readers the kinds of day-to-day middle-class mental and physical abuses which were widely believed to encourage the introduction of disease. The range of abuse worried instructors more than any specific vice. To be sure, they were very concerned with masturbation and sexual overemployment, but few were obsessive on individual issues. Historians have tended to overfocus on masturbation. To avoid ill health, one should banish "excessive indulgence of the emotions . . . frantic, desultory efforts to accomplish in one hour an amount of mental work appropriate to double the amount of time. . . . Attempting to do two things at one and the same time . . . [or] petty social or other arrangements which interfere with the function of sleep . . . constipation . . . [stuffing with] rich, indigestible food."[5] A glance at a late nineteenth-century restaurant menu lends credence to the connection between overeating and certain forms of sickness,

45

but warnings against expressing violent emotions were even more frequent. Excesses even of positive feelings such as mirth and joy, as well as sexual desire, could lead to discord, as would, even more certainly, such negative passions as fear, hatred, jealousy, and anger.[6] Even repression could be immoderate, as in the discussion of sexual continence which we address in chapter 5. A calm equilibrium was the desired norm in a society recently wracked by civil war and presently rent by industrial and urban confrontations.

In this commonsense framework, disease was the result of basic transgressions from law, that is, departures from an attainable and sustainable moderation of behavior. This almost amounted to a covenant theory of health: if the individual avoided immoderation, he or she would be rewarded with freedom from disease. Thus was the justice of nature made less blind and harsh. Perhaps it was this line of thought which led to such a Mosaic title as *The Ten Laws of Health,* by J. R. Black, who argued that bad health was not due to external forces or to bad blood since each human being started fresh, regardless of what his ancestors had done, and could choose the rewards of lawfulness or the punishments of lawlessness. But God, of course, had toyed with His chosen people, and a lifetime in the wilderness seemed only too possible in the world of late nineteenth-century American health.

Disease and health were also interpreted as interrelated parts of a natural whole. In fact, disease symptoms could be seen as signposts of the recovery of the body from sickly states. Such a notion was based upon the theory of vitalism, an ageless belief reformulated in the late eighteenth and nineteenth centuries in a variety of etiologies and therapies. Disease, rather than being a force external to the body, was a derangement of the vital principles which operated the body from within. Although appearing to take differing forms, disease actually had only one cause. As an imbalance, disease could be eliminated when the vital, natural tendencies of the body were activated again to restore its equilibrium. Here again, nature was presumably beneficent.[7]

The predominant application of vitalism in late nineteenth-century America remained homeopathy, a theory of European origin which had been attractive to many Americans since the late eighteenth century. Unlike regular medics with their heroic and sometimes fatal dosages and purges, homeopathists used small dosages of medicine which were intended to heighten in the human body the disease symptoms already present. Such medication would further the effectiveness of the already engaged disease-repelling mechanism in the body. One homeopath described his science to the readers of *Popular Science Monthly* in 1893: "Homeopathy, as a science, is the law of the vital force; the body is but the mechanism upon which it operates . . . disease is the impairment of the equalization of vital force, and it finds expression where the organism is weakest. . . . To cure is to locate the center of the disturbance . . . and to restore the equilibrium. As there is but one nerve-center of a disease, so there is but one remedy."[8]

Homeopathy was but the most widespread therapeutic application of vitalist theories in late nineteenth-century America. Hydropathists believed that the ingestion of pure water and submersion in it (often adjoined to a general asceticism) would allow the body to spring back to its natural resilience. The water cure, one hydropath insisted, would be the central means to help along bodily restoration. "All diseases are remedial efforts, whose object is the defense and purification of the vital organism, and the reparation of the deranged structure."[9] Other therapists believed that the vital component of the body was electrical and that applications of small doses of galvanic energy from electrical batteries would therefore lead the body to recharge itself. "Disease of every character . . . originates in a derangement of the circulation of vital electricity," wrote a popular health writer whose methods of electrical therapies were shared by some regular physicians as well.[10]

Disequilibrium, the overloading of one or another circuit, was a danger implicit not merely in electrical therapy, but in all vitalist conceptions of the body, where disease and health were parts of a whole. Hence humans were responsible for maintaining the vital balance, and could, through immoderate behavior, tip the bodily scales toward disease. "On this principle, [if] any class of organs or any part of the body be unduly . . . exercised, it requires the more nutrition to support them, thereby withdrawing what should go to the other organs."[11] One of the more obvious of such dissipations centered on the genitals of adolescents, a subject to which we will return.[12] Contrarily, vitalism also implied that vital energies could be focused on specific bodily deficiencies, thereby restoring balance: "Within certain limits, the nervous fluid or vital force strengthens and develops any part of the body or brain in proportion as it is brought to bear upon it."[13] Care had to be taken, however, to avoid excessive corrective focusing lest the "cure" create its own disease.

Vitalist thinkers were in harmony with much mid to late nineteenth-century medical thought in their insistence that disruptions within the body, rather than unknown external factors, caused illness. It was a matter of pride to many physicians that they no longer looked at disease as a "visitation," inscrutable and unremovable. The eminent physician Samuel W. Gross, writing in 1887 of his fifty years in medicine, commented that when he had entered the profession "it was overspread with a mantle of darkness. . . . Hardly anything was definitely settled. . . . Disease was by many regarded, not as an aberration of function, or perversion of health, but as a sort of undefinable entity engrafted upon the system, from which it was necessary to expel it, often with violent remedies, more injurious to the patient than the malady itself."[14] What Gross did not acknowledge or did not know was that mere ignorance alone had not led American physicians to use vigorous actions to rid the body of foreign contaminants. Strong assaults had been part of the claim of newly independent Americans that theirs was an innovative country needing special rules and customs. American disease, more incapacitating and lethal than the European disorders on which the first textbooks had been based, required, in this view, prompt and decisive action.[15]

By the 1870s, the emphasis on disruptions within the body, which had succeeded the external factors as an explanation for disease, itself became inadequate as an etiological system. In health issues, as in other aspects of American life, insistence upon the sanctity and independence of the individual clashed with increasing collectivization and interdependency. It was no longer possible to ignore completely the impact of external factors upon the health of the individual. No matter how much health writers talked about imbalances, disruptions, and immoderation, they could not banish that whole series of forces which lay outside individual control. The public health movement, which dated in America from mid-century, was built on the idea that whole populations, affected by epidemic outbreaks of infectious disease, could be defended only with collective hygienic measures. It was difficult, however, to give up the notion of varying vulnerability to disease among individuals. Neither a strictly contagionist nor a purely miasmatist (putrified air and water as the cause of disease) position could explain why some people contracted yellow fever when others did not. Therefore, the most widely held theoretical view, according to George Rosen, a leading twentieth-century historian of public health, combined parts of both theories: infectious diseases were due to contagia which could not act except in conjunction with other elements such as the state of the atmosphere, condition of the soil, and social factors such as urban crowding.[16] Such a formulation, which combined biological and social factors, also allowed room for emphasis upon the condition of the individual as recipient or resister to epidemics.

The reception given the new science of bacteriology at the end of the period we are discussing provides a clear illustration both of the lack of consensus as to the ultimate causes and subsequent definitions of disease and of a deep urge to hold individuals responsible for their own state of health. The isolation of specific bacilli for a wide range of human and animal diseases in the 1880s and 1890s presented the possibility that diseases were uncontrollable invasions from hostile forces which lay in nature outside the body. Indeed, many American physicians resisted the germ theory because its refined explanation of the causes of disease initially was of no aid to them in the actual treatment of their patients.[17] Contrarily, the popular reception of bacteriology was more positive, possibly because many individuals felt that they could share the burden of their own responsibility for disease with invisible armies of invaders (just as they tried to shift blame for social disruption onto the new immigrants). In 1885, Henry Thompson, writing in *Popular Science Monthly,* attributed much of the growing interest in medicine to ready public acceptance of bacteriology: "The germ theory appeals to the average mind: it is something tangible; it may be hunted down, captured, colored, and looked at through a microscope, and then in all its varieties, it can be held directly responsible for so much damage. There is scarcely a farmer in the country who has not read of the germ-theory. A cow-boy in Arizona was shot dead in the saddle recently by a comrade for the insult implied by calling him a 'd——d microbe!' " Some physicians themselves were not immune from squeamishness at the actual sight of microorganisms under the microscope, although to one fastidious Kansas doctor, seeing was finally believing. He witnessed with "repulsive interest" the "hidious animaculae that live and moved and grew in a drop of Neosho water." Since seeing "fat thousand-legged bugs retreating from a particle of a prune placed under the microscope," Dr. J. J. Wright "excluded this fruit from his bill of fare" and resolved to keep his other favorite foods away from the magnifying lens lest "mere existence would seem so hazardous that life itself would become burdensome."[18] Perhaps this was the microscopic equivalent to the awful Victorian fascination with the machine in the garden. In the popular reception of bacteriology, there was no apparent interest in distinguishing one bacillus from another; consequently, already popular panaceas became increasingly attractive. James Harvey Young describes the career of William Radom, who, in the 1880s, made his fortune from his

Microbe Killer, proclaimed by its promoter to be a universal antiseptic, which when taken in large amounts would infiltrate all the tissues and blood but would kill only bacteria and any other diseases that happened to be present.[19]

For a period after 1870, many bacteriologists themselves viewed pathogenic microorganisms as the single and complete cause of disease, if not as disease itself. In this sense was disease once again an external entity visited upon the body.[20] However, by the 1880s, the sovereign role of bacilli had been reduced to that of a causal factor, interrelated with bodily responses to them. In the language of one physician writing in 1883, disease was "the struggle between the parasitic invaders and the animal cells . . . parasites are not the disease, but only its cause. The disease itself is an alteration of the physiological processes, as a response to some unwonted influence."[21] Through such a formulation it was possible to reintroduce human responsibility for disease. One had internal resources, whether mental, moral, or behavioral, to marshal against the dreadful invaders. Even a Christian Scientist could incorporate bacteriology within his world view: "The bacteria revealed by the microscope have no power to infect the body unless the mind consents."[22]

Bacteriology, although containing the seeds of pessimism concerning human vulnerability to disease, by century's end lent itself to a more positive understanding. Hereditarianism, by contrast, remained a gloomy variable in the explanation of disease. Unlike the other levels of explanation for disease we have discussed, hereditarianism by the 1870s was based on an almost totally negative determinism: forces outside of and antedating the life of individuals would fundamentally shape them, their proclivity to disease, their recuperative ability, in ways probably beyond their control. In an equally negative sense, hereditarianism was applied to the American social scene to explain the fatuity of attempting to integrate alien nationalities and races into the civilized mainstream. Just as the inherited forces tending toward health and vitality were ignored, so were positive "permanent" characteristics of foreigners and blacks who were declared irrelevant to the American mix. Charles Rosenberg has argued convincingly that the transition from optimism to pessimism in regard to social hereditarianism that occurred from the mid-nineteenth century on was not provoked by any substantial changes in the body of pertinent scientific knowledge.[23] If Americans increasingly saw individual sickness and antisocial behavior as strictly controlled by hereditary factors, it was not because scientific findings pushed them to these conclusions, but rather because their fears about what was happening in the social sector made such interpretations especially compelling.

Hereditarian code words such as *survival of the fittest, degeneracy,* and *abnormal variations* indicated that within humankind lay the seeds of inevitable decay. Here, justice would mean only punishment. Even a normally optimistic physician could conclude that "the laws of hereditary descent are the most potent of all the influences that determine the character and destinies of individuals and of nations. Climate and diet, powerful as they are, must always yield to unconquerable might of race, and can of themselves work only incidental and transient changes in the original types." He went on to stress that "every quality of organic existence tends to be hereditary . . . that all vices of the system may be transmitted."[24] Eugenicists often laid down a far harsher line of conclusions. Some found it possible almost to celebrate the death of inferior stock from disease. For example, one writer in *Popular Science Monthly* depicted high infant mortality as a just and natural screening mechanism. Explaining which children succumbed to the common diseases of infancy, he declared in an updated ideological equivalent of the Calvinist doctrine of infant damnation that "a very large proportion of all children born into the world are either weaklings or invalids from the beginning." Physical, moral, and racial fitness were here all parts of a whole, and the nonsurvival of the unfit a merciful provision. "A race of criminals, paupers, and idiots deteriorates with each successive generation and goes down to speedy extinction."[25]

The same underlying hope, that inferior people would

automatically die as a result of their flawed constitutions, permeated the thinking of less overtly eugenicist writers as well. It
is only by this interpretation that we can make sense of the occa-
sional defeatist warnings which seemed to release people from
responsibility for their own health. "About two-thirds of our
people inherit a tendency to some disease or to a defective vitality
in some organ of the body. . . . Those defectively organized
cannot overstep the bounds of the most watchful prudence without incurring suffering. Only by the most minute and accurate
knowledge of hygiene, and unswerving attention to its require-
ments, are they enabled to avoid pain, disease and an untimely
death."[26] In this advice, written in 1879, which was in contrast to
the urgings of many other advisors from this and earlier periods
to struggle against any inherited constitutional bent toward specific diseases, pain, disease, and a horrible fate seem much more
likely than the meager prevention that even the most watchful
behavior could provide. Did the writer of these words, J. R. Black,
who had earlier in the decade promised good health in exchange
for following ten simple laws, seriously expect his readers to
forswear enjoyment and ease for the single-minded, joyless, even
immoderate, regimen apparently required not even to assure
good health, but just to ward off disaster? Might not the reader
just as easily conclude not to bother striving for the paltry reward? That, in fact, was the message of another author who wrote
in the same journal, *Popular Science Monthly,* a decade later. Black
did not state specifically who the better endowed one-third of the
population was: Clement Hammond, associate editor of the Boston *Globe,* from his survey of New England farmers and their
wives, concluded that it was these light-complexioned folks of
sanguine-nervous temperament who were most prone to longevity. Their regular, moderate habits were not the cause of their
good health and long lives, but were yet another expression of
their temperaments. He dismissed as peripheral: sanitary conditions, simple, easily digestible food, complete abstinence from
stimulants and tobacco. "Given a certain organization of mind
and body," Hammond concluded, "I think that a man can count

on long life—always barring accidents—with reasonable certainty."[27] The covert message of these two authors was that certain people by nature of their inherited constitutions were so flawed as to make any prophylactic or reparative efforts useless in their struggle to survive. Those who were meant, by their temperaments and builds and genetic inheritence, to flourish and carry on, would do so. At the foundation of this reasoning ran the belief in continued white Anglo-Saxon Protestant domination: native-born Americans might not be able to keep foreigners out, nor to outbreed them, but they would certainly outlast them, and in so doing, prevail. In this secularized, scientific fashion, the ideal of a racial elect might be preserved, and the gloomiest predestinarianism might yet yield a kind of comfort, at least among those readers who were of the chosen stock.

Hereditarianism was the ideological form within which the most negative present and future for the errant individual was expressed. Here disease was destiny for all but a predetermined few. However, we do not mean to imply by the structure of this chapter that hereditarian thought was the culmination of all late nineteenth-century writing about disease. On the contrary, most health instructors believed, as we have shown, that natural justice was potentially beneficent as well as destructive, and that sensible men and women should struggle perpetually to avoid or overcome most diseases and lead healthy lives. Such a stance was consistent, after all, with the genre in which they chose to write. Hereditarianism is, nevertheless, the most unambiguous demonstration that optimism about mankind's redeemable fate existed in an ongoing and perhaps losing contest with negative potentialities, with the punishing face of justice. And yet, more ambiguous ideological strands, such as those presented by reworked vitalism, held out some hope, and the implications of the most negative determinism were probably not understood in a systematic fashion. Even in much hereditarian presentation, to say nothing of its reception, capitulation into passive despair did not seem to follow determinism.

54

4

Brain and
Mind in Sickness
and in Health

In contexts other than hereditarianism, determinism sometimes contained more unequivocally hopeful applications. Seeking to establish themselves as the legitimate experts on the mind and to find solid bases on which to treat insanity, late nineteenth-century neurophysiologists found materialist definitions of the mind to be distinctly liberating. The brain, they declared, was the organ of the mind, and it was only through study of the brain that the mind could be explored. No longer must students of the mind be trapped in the misty morality of the metaphysicians; they knew now that measurable physiological changes defined the health of the mind. Relegated to superstitious bigotry of less advanced times was the notion that insanity was a visitation from the devil. "So long as the mind was regarded as something separated from the body, or only united to it by feeble ties, bodily conditions could have nothing to do with mental phenomena—insanity was a disease of the soul," a prominent British physiologist reminded the readers of *Popular Science Monthly* in 1875. "The monk, standing over a miserable lunatic chained to a staple in the wall, and flogging him in order to make him cast his devil out was a logical outcome of this hypothesis. . . . The advent of physiological psychology is at hand. [Insanity] is now known to be linked with appreciable pathological changes, and in many instances is amenable to physical remedial agents." This same writer then gave a rather typical late nineteenth-century physiologically materialist definition of thought: "Thought is the product of the cells of the grey matter of the brain—the result of a change of form in inorganic matter taken into the system as food."[1]

In attempting to free "mental physics" from metaphysics, neurophysiologists tended to reinforce a bipolarity: the physicality of the actions of the brain as opposed to the ethereality of consciousness. As a later generation of behavioral psychologists would do in a somewhat parallel manner, late nineteenth-century neurophysiologists then tended to conclude that only chemical and physical brain changes and specific functions of particular centers in the brain could be explored experimentally and rationally. Since consciousness (or as many of them would have put it, the mind, or even the soul) was, by its nature, unamenable to scientific exploration, it was therefore to be dismissed as a subject for direct investigation, only to be dealt with, sometime in the future, as derivative from brain processes. "To the metaphysician, mind is an independent entity in an upper sphere of being," E. L. Youmans, an American scientific popularizer, wrote with barely concealed scorn in 1882. "To the mental physiologist, it is the activity of an organized mass of nerve-cells and filaments, charged with blood and carrying on processes of thinking and feeling under the laws of nutrition."[2]

The chief thrust of physiological research was in isolating the locus of functions in specific brain regions. Most such localization study, carried on at the time chiefly in Germany, France, and England on laboratory animals, met a positive response in

America, partly due to widespread fascination, dating back to the 1830s, with phrenology. Through studying and classifying configurations of the skull, phrenologists believed that they were studying mind only as it made itself manifest in precise physical forms. Mind or character traits, both those largely and those insufficiently developed, originated in a larger or smaller area of the brain and skull. Thus many believed that phrenology could provide a scientific base for the determination and education of character. By 1880, phrenologists could feel that the new localization studies confirmed the main thrust of their beliefs. "The results of a course of such [localization] experiments which have been published . . . are exceedingly interesting to the student of Phrenology, because they constitute a physical demonstration of the fact that the brain is an assemblage of centers subserving distinct functions."[3] On their part, the new neurophysiologists understood the contributions as well as the limitations of phrenology. They believed that only brain structure affected mind and that elevations on the skull were irrelevant, but they also believed that phrenologists, in searching for a physical basis of mind, had been on the right track. "We are indebted to the phrenological school for having made a vigorous fight on behalf of the claims of the head upon the students of the mind, and whatever may be the imperfections of their scheme, they have actually cleared away a vast amount of prejudice in the popular mind, and prepared for the consideration of the material apparatus in connection with mental phenomena."[4]

Although they rejected the skull for the organ inside, many neurophysiologists were as literal about measurements in their attempts to derive mind from brain. Dating from the mid nineteenth century, and still a topic of discussion in serious journals in the 1880s, was the attempt to establish average brain sizes and weights as the way to quantify intelligence, an evidently useful means to sort out and rank increasingly heterogeneous populations and occupational orders in a society which disavowed aristocracy. Usually, calculations confirmed the social status quo with northern European males on the top, southern

Europeans and women well down the list, and blacks on the bottom. In 1880, for example, H. Hughes Bennett wrote in *Popular Science Monthly* that "as the organ of intellect in the female is smaller and lighter than that in the male, we may fairly assume that it is less capable of high and extended mental powers."[5] By 1887, Joseph Simms, also writing in *Popular Science Monthly,* was still painstakingly measuring brain weights, but was more fascinated with the disparities between brain size and intelligence than with their congruence. "While intelligence is rapidly increasing from twenty to sixty years of age, the brain is diminishing. The time that a man knows most is from seventy to eighty, but then his brain is smaller than when he was a little boy between seven and fourteen, the age when he thought he knew the most."[6]

With the aid of a tradition of materialist views of the brain, and with a new experimental method, many scientists anticipated that in the future they would be able to "picture a physical base of nerve cells, joined together by nerve fibers, so that it seems probable that the mechanism of thought will someday be understood." It was presumed in this argument that "physical conditions [would] determine mental results" and that the study of the brain tissues would reduce thought to "transformed energy" which would thus have a "physiological representation and measurable force." Not content with localization studies on higher animals, one prominent American neurologist, influenced by the cries of *"Ohne Phosphor, kein Gedanke"* coming from Germany in the 1860s, believed that one could measure at least the degree of human mind exertion by analyzing wastes from thought in the physical form of urine contents. "As a chemist, by weighing the ashes on the hearth, determines how much wood has been burnt, so the physiologist, by weighing the ashes of the brain—the phosphates—measures the amount of thought."[7]

The phrenologists were perfectionist materialists who had believed that their science would evoke the maximum potential in each human brain; the new physiologists, on the other hand, in keeping with the diminished optimism concerning human potential after mid-century, rarely mentioned brain improvement as the outcome of their method. The primary application of their form of materialism was in the realm of pathology—the definition and etiology of insanity—and in brain surgery. Typically, neurophysiological definitions of insanity assumed that mental disintegration followed physical breakdown of the brain. "Insanity is a term applied to certain results of brain disease and brain defect which invalidate integrity." "Physiological perversions are causes of mental derangement." "[Insanity] is a disorder of the supreme nerve-centers of the brain."[8] In all three of these definitions, the neurophysiologists were careful to stress that insanity was a disease in the same sense as any other. "A disordered mind is as surely the result of a disordered brain," yet another authority asserted, "as dyspepsia is of a deranged stomach."[9] But what if the correct analogy were to stomach cancer and not to dyspepsia? Some physiologists were driven to this logical and gloomy conclusion, which also had the advantage of being clear-cut. "Starting from the point that all normal mental phenomena are the result of the action of a healthy brain, and that all abnormal manifestations of the mind are the result of the functioning of a diseased or deranged brain, I do not see why the latter should not be included under the designation of 'insanity', as much as the former are embraced under the term 'sanity.' " William A. Hammond, a surgeon who became an alienist, then relentlessly concluded, "There can be no middle ground, for the brain is either in a healthy or an unhealthy condition. If healthy, the product of its action is 'sanity;' if unhealthy, 'insanity.' "[10]

If, following this line of reasoning, insanity were a purely physical cerebral decadence, the causes of this material result were not so clear to the neurophysiologists. Changes in the reflex action of the nervous system or in the blood supply or in the composition of the bile or urine would be the mediating factors which would lead to brain alteration. But what events would lead to a pathological condition in the mediating factors? Here materialist neurophysiology overlapped with nonmaterial causation. Whereas a sudden introduction of cocaine, for example, or an abrupt digestive breakdown could still be seen as physical causes of material results in the brain, emotional and moral causes were often considered the real culprits, somehow triggering material events. Hence, one neurophysiologist's list of the causes of insanity would include categories such as diabetes and irregular secretions of the glands alongside categories such as melancholy and obsession with work. This same writer published an article in *Popular Science Monthly* entitled "Induced Disease From the Influence of the Passions," in which he blended moral and physiological causes: "Whenever from undue excitement of any kind, the passions are permitted to overrule the reason, the result is disease: the heart empties itself into the brain, the brain is stricken, the heart is prostrate and both are lost." Many writers wanted to believe that as in the case of physical disorders, responsibility for mental disease was finally in the hands of the individual who could induce, through bad acts habitually repeated, deterioration of the brain. Through good habits, on the other hand, he or she could maintain a healthy brain.[11]

There were no available mechanisms by which to measure physiological brain deterioration in the living, so for late nineteenth-century Americans, behavior was the only available indication of the state of the brain. Definitions of insanity were arrived at, then as now, through social consensus evaluating appropriate behavior. William A. Hammond's insistence that, physiologically considered, the brain produced either sane or insane actions did not permit of that whole range of behavior that appeared neither totally healthy nor definitely sick. Although a few of the grievously insane met the traditional legal definition of not being able to distinguish right from wrong, there were many more who were able to tell right from wrong, but were unable or unwilling to do right, and thus were insane according to many doctors. This was, in the terms of the times, *moral insanity*. Moral insanity, as the modern historian Norman Dain defines it, was "an individual's emotional inability to accept society's judgments about anti-social actions."[12]

Contemporary observers saw many people as being insane

on some subjects but not at all on others. In this way, as in the use of moral insanity, sanity and insanity became less categorical functionally. "There is no definite line where sanity ends and insanity begins. The question of insanity is simply a question of degree. . . . All disease is partial disease; until we reach death, we are partly well."[13] To make mental categories less rigid was to accept some degree of disorder not only in personal lives but also in the body politic. Americans were having to learn to live with their own political and social tendencies to lawlessness without dismissing themselves as complete failures. Rather than aiming for a total moral and communal harmony, such assessments, coming after a devastatingly disruptive Civil War, suggest the more modest goals of maintaining personal and social equilibrium.

Observers of behavior muted physiological clarity in the popularly disseminated definitions of insanity. Still, as in all societies, lines were drawn between those considered hopelessly insane and those who could be cured. In late nineteenth-century America, the category of the hopelessly insane who were to be locked away was larger than it had been in antebellum America. In the 1830s and 1840s, "moral therapy" was a perfectionist ideology used for curing the deranged. As Gerald N. Grob has vividly shown, the cure rates apparently were a great deal higher in mid nineteenth-century America, when moral therapists believed they could cure mental disease, and their patients gained strength from positive therapy, than in the late ninteenth century, when many psychiatrists believed that positive therapy was improbable where physiological decay, whatever its ultimate causes, was outside of human capability to correct. Furthermore, many of the late nineteenth-century insane were new immigrants with whom the therapists could not identify. Concerns about insanity and with the new immigrations of eastern and southern Europeans meshed in the minds of late nineteenth-century nativists.[14]

If severe insanity was nearly impossible to cure in practice, it became important to establish lines between the hopelessly insane and those who could respond to treatment. Apparently, increasing numbers of newly urbanized Americans, natives and immigrants alike, suffered from an inability to function adequately or happily within their social roles, exhibiting symptoms of mild depression, of what one late nineteenth-century physician observed to be "nervous debility and irritability." In 1881, this physician, George M. Beard, characterized such a state as "nervousness," and this became a widely accepted definition of what we now call neurosis. In part, Beard was eager, as were other physicians, to distinguish nervousness from psychosis in order to maintain a large area for positive therapy. "Although nervousness sometimes leads to insanity . . . yet there is no necessary correlation between simple nervousness and the extreme or special manifestation of it in the form of insanity. Thousands and thousands are nervous who are not and never will be insane."[15] Rest and insulation from the irritations of normal social intercourse were the basic components of the various therapies applied to "nervous" individuals. The most elaborate and well-known therapy of the late nineteenth century was that of S. Weir Mitchell, who concentrated upon distraught upper middle-class women. Mitchell sealed off his patients in a large bed chamber, crammed them with vast amounts of rich, nourishing food, sedated them into deep and prolonged sleep, and kept them away as completely as possible from all their usual, frustrating social contacts, the better to soothe them with his own calm presence.[16] Therapies such as Mitchell's commanded a return to a kind of childlike dependency and regularity as the base point of psychic reconstruction.

In an industrializing society in which an increasing proportion of the population was engaged in sedentary brain work rather than in physical labor, advisors focused much attention on brain and mind. One somewhat extreme statement highlights the preoccupation with mental activities and problems. Burt G. Wilder believed that human evolution had occurred in just the last century, for, as he explained, men just one hundred years earlier had been larger, coarser, lustier by nature, having "less brain and more blood." By 1875, people's bodies were no longer the basic, organic problem, but their brains, and most especially their imaginations, were decided causes for concern.[17] Insanity, nervousness, brain overwork, and brain size were all issues which provoked controversy and called for causal explanations relating to the peculiarities of American society at that time. Social causation was never really absent from late nineteenth-century analysis of organically centered insanity, and it was given a yet larger role in explanations of nervousness: "This is the nervous age of the world's history." Those awesome forces which lent modern civilization its power also tended to overwhelm the ability of individuals to assimilate and master their new conditions. The fear that civilization and its lures induced physical disorders also applied to mental health. The ironic mixture of awe and despair which characterized the gaze of Henry Adams upon the dynamo was not an isolated view of "social progress." George Beard, too, looked upon the symbols of modern culture—"steam power, the periodical press, the telegraph, the sciences, and the mental activity of women"—and saw in these expressions of new ways of approaching the world and of making a living the "chief and primary cause of this development and very rapid increase of nervousness in modern civilization."[18] Late nineteenth-century America engendered harsh problems for the aspiring individual. As opposed to an earlier social homogeneity, wrote one therapist, American society was now characterized by "dissonance" and "struggle for existence" due to "alienated interests" of various new industrial social classes. In addition (and with unintentional contradiction), this writer continued with the thought that American democratic institutions and lack of an identifiable privileged class "lends a morbid impetuosity to the efforts of both the poor and moderately rich members of the community, to attempt to climb the mentally exhausting ladder to success."[19]

It was upon the new middle class in particular that nervousness was visited. In the statement of purpose for the founding of *The Journal of Nervous and Mental Disease* in 1874, J. S. Jewell, the editor, explained that the new and increasing "sedentary and mental occupations . . . exhaust the power and augment the sensibilities of the nervous system, or tend to destroy a healthy equilibrium between the development and action of the nervous, as compared with other systems of the body."[20] The self-discipline required for these occupations, tied to apparent opportunity for upward mobility, imposed a mighty strain on the psyches of the new middle classes. As we have suggested already, beneath the surface lurked anxiety concerning the rhythms, the meaning, the validity of these new occupations whose relation to production was somewhat hazy. And yet to survive, it was not fruitful to have such doubts. Emotional sublimation linked to intellectual striving could lead to an overwhelming mental conflict, which worried the analysts of the new nervousness. Beard warned, "One cause of the increase of nervous diseases is that the conventionalities of society require the emotions to be repressed, while the activity of our civilization gives an unprecedented freedom and opportunity for the expression of the intellect; the more we feel, the more we must restrain our feelings."[21] One result of this anguish produced by increases in mental strain was the problem, new to late nineteenth-century Americans, of drug abuse. Sufferers turned to drugs when the technological developments of the hypodermic syringe and the derivation of morphine from opium coincided with the inability of physicians to offer other generally effective remedies for physical and mental pain.[22] In the opinion of carefully nonmoralistic late nineteenth-century observers, alcoholism, the traditional form of drug abuse which cut across class lines, continued to flourish as another compensation for this stress.

Not merely did intolerable mental strain lead to degenerative cravings and nervousness, but what was more dangerous, it was destroying the potential for the development of children. Late nineteenth-century educators and physicians were enormously concerned with what they called "brain exhaustion." The teaching of basic skills and moral truths had begun to give way, under the technical demands of industrial society, to intensive study of specialized information, leading, they felt, to "brain-forcing"—overintellectualization, subdivision of knowledge, and cramming. New, artificial production demanded new, artificial education. "The mind is treated [by educators] as a kind of general receptacle into which knowledge almost indiscriminately must be poured, yes forced," one physician declared. This "unnatural" forcing would lead away from that "harmony and complete development of all parts of the brain," which had been the goal of character-training educators, and toward "an excessive development of the nervous temperament." Such misdirected mental growth might well put the student on the road to "irritability and morbidness," bad mental habits which would frequently lead to brain disease and the lunatic asylum.[23] Hard study would wear out the body more than physical labor, ran a typical warning in a popular magazine. Under these conditions the brain would receive a disproportionate amount of blood.[24]

Blood supply and nerve force were, in fact, analagous and almost interchangeable metaphors for the life-enhancing, vital forces in the body and the mind. This had particular meaning for the education of girls beyond the three R's into high school and university training. If the basic function of women was as reproducers of the race, then why educate them in the same way as men, asked Dr. Edward H. Clarke, a member of the Harvard Board of Overseers who wished to keep women out of that university. His book *Sex in Education, or a Fair Chance for the Girls* was a runaway best seller, around which flourished a swirl of controversy. Clarke's basic argument was that the "catamenial function" in adolescent girls could not be properly established if their teachers diverted force to the brain that was needed elsewhere. "The system never does two things well at the same time," he warned. As one of his supporters put it, her education continues unabated throughout the month, forcing the girl to use, during her menstrual period, "a large part of the nerve-force which should be directed to the genital organs, and she is exhausted by the effort of carrying on two processes at once."[25] This fear that young women were being diverted from their real work as mothers, at a time of rapidly dropping birth rates, especially among the more educated, is but a more explicit formulation of the general worry that brain work of uncertain suitability was superseding more clearly productive labor in importance. Just as a disproportionate amount of energy in the bodily economy was being directed toward the brain and away from physical development, so were the energies of middle-class Americans being focused toward work requiring mental skills rather than physical labor.

Not everyone shared this concern, however; some were more optimistic about people's adaptation to these changes. A whole anti-Clarke faction emerged, particularly among women physicians, maintaining that women could and did manage study and menstruation simultaneously without endangering themselves or the perpetuation of the race.[26] There were also those who chafed against the general preoccupation with brain exhaustion. Mental sloth was as great a danger as mental overwork, they claimed. The brain, like all other parts of the body, their argument ran, crumbled under an unaccustomed work load and needed to become "habituated to the constant gymnastic influence of steady work." Healthy thinking had not merely to be "systematic and consecutive," but positive, not "in a downward direction, which fret, worry, mar and sear" the self, but "in an upward course." George Beard, the great explainer of American nervousness, was on balance also the reassurer of urban white-collar workers. He explained to them why they were nervous, informed them that nervousness was a physical state with comprehensible causes, and assured them that humans someday would find a balance between the sensible and insensible, and that by extension, their children would not turn out to be puny and distraught creatures.[27] In the meantime, whether they were optimists or pessimists about the long-range outcome of the impact of modernity, advisors, by their acknowledgment that contemporary life could be difficult, were giving permission for their readers to seek treatment for their anguish without feeling guilty or self-indulgent, and were justifying the work of new mental therapists such as Mitchell or Beard.

As in the case of physical illness, the advisors pondered the causes of brain and mind dysfunction, assessed the impact of what they termed *modern civilization,* argued whether a *natural* way of living could be reconstructed to promote mental health, and ended, here, too, by developing a hygiene about brain exhaustion which answered no fundamental questions, but which filled the hunger for self-determination and predictability. For instance, many educators felt that a discoverable set of hygienic laws existed which, when correctly applied, would overcome brain exhaustion and even the general cultural tendency toward nervousness. "When our educators become thoroughly convinced that physical development as a part of education is an absolute necessity—that a strict observance of the laws of physiology and hygiene is indispensable to the highest mental culture —then we shall have vital and radical changes in our educational system."[28] The structure of the school day could be correlated to the laws of body chemistry. Intense study should occur in the morning "when the brain is refreshed and repaired by a night's repose." After lunch, when the blood supply was presumed to be focused in the stomach rather than in the brain, lighter subjects were appropriate. Recess periods should follow times of concentration. Most important, well-rounded physical education was the chief reformist means to counterbalance brainwork.[29] Similar hygienic measures were appropriate for adults. Exercise for them would redirect the blood supply, relieving the brain of congestion. Sound sleep, which would "repair damage and clear away debris," could compensate for heavy brain use during the day. Thus a corrective rhythm could be established: whereas "during the hours of wakefulness the destruction of brain-tissue exceeds the nutrition . . . during sleep the ganglia hoard up an amount of available explosive energy."[30] Once again, in this argument, the natural balances essential to health had been destroyed by civilization, and it was necessary for the individual to establish conscious forms of behavior to compensate for the lost instincts.

Emphasis on brain exhaustion, in particular, and nervousness, in general, exemplified the assumption that the supply of vital force or energy in humans was finite and that overexpenditure in one activity would tax the body or the mind in other processes. This sense of a limited energy pool was a kind of mercantilism of self. Although in the next chapters we will show that this assumption had application in the sexual sphere as well, it was a pervasive belief about all the functions of the body and the mind. In this mercantilist framework, the limited fund of resources meant that each usage depleted the fund. "In the great economy of nature force answers to force and everything must be paid for. . . . The writing of this work, of this paragraph, of this very sentence, costs more or less cerebral substance, which if not replaced will leave the author poorer than when he began it." Given the materialist neurophysiological assumptions which we have described, it followed that "there is a limit to our acquiring power, and this is largely determined by . . . the size of the brain." Hence there was not room in the brain for all knowledge, and "if we acquire more we must forget something we already know." Selective forgetfulness had to match selective acquisition. Beard used a vivid metaphor to make the point to the victims of nervousness he saw all about him: "The brain is a hotel where the words make but a short stay, or perhaps stop but for a night, then pass on; were they to become permanent guests the space would be at once overcrowded, and there would be no room for newcomers."[31] Even genius, which would seem to imply a brain less limited than most, was for some advisors yet another example of the finite quality of the human brain, and the dangers of immoderation of all sorts. Martin Luther Holbrook characterized great genius as a "nervous disease," and surmised that "it can only exist where all the nervous tissue is occupied with one class of thoughts to the exclusion of another class, both of which are necessary to mental health."[32] Holbrook's antiintellectual leveling was not unusual in a culture in which the all-around citizen was still the democratic norm, despite the economic and social necessity for increasingly intensive intellectual and technical training in high schools and colleges, and not merely for geniuses.

Employers of the late nineteenth-century mercantilist analogy envisioned an ideal corporeal state in which "waste and repair compensate one another in a rhythmic balance." In this ideal state, only correct uses of the body could balance strenuous uses of the mind. Modern urban life, especially for the middle classes, ran contrary to this ideal. There, observers feared, "excessive intellectual activity often produces a weak state of the system." Modern civilization warped some natural equilibrium which had presumably existed in premodern culture. "In highly civilized communities," J. S. Jewell worried, "there is a constant tendency to a loss of balance in nerve development, in which the sensitive side of the nervous system preponderates over the motor part." The mercantilist analogy was part of the larger analysis of the social causes of nervousness. Evidently, Jewell concluded, civilization "carries with it the causes or condition of decay." Perhaps the psyches of individuals would be overwhelmed by an imperious and impossible cultural milieu, ultimately more damaging than any overt violence done to the body: "The nervous system is the part of the organism which is to be the chief theatre of the ruin with which the race . . . seems likely to be overtaken."[33] Individuals appeared trapped in a double causal web. On the one hand, neurophysiological materialism led to the conclusion that large, perhaps controlling, portions of brain function were outside of personal control. On the other hand, modern civilization seemed to be inducing insuperable mental strain. Good behavior, always necessary, led to only a limited self-determination at best.

5

Making
Sense
of Sex

B oth the physiological matrix and modern civilization, as late nineteenth-century Americans perceived them, produced limitations on the self which threatened to be overwhelming. Yet by no means did defeatism follow. Striving for positive self-definition was presumed to be the obligation of the good individual. This struggle was a serious matter, for it occurred in a cultural arena of limiting and perhaps finally overpowering forces. Apparently, one had only finite personal energy in a world in which endless demands were made on that energy at home, at the workplace, in schools, in the whirligig of cities and towns.

This point reemerged through whatever metaphor was chosen to describe the human energy supply. The mercantilist image of available energy was not one of hoarding a surplus or stimulating growth of one's resources, but rather, of maintaining one's scarce fund of goods. Energy, talent, beauty, intelligence —all these resources were limited and in danger of depletion and ultimate exhaustion. A sense of imminent loss was more characteristic of this image of energy than was greed for more and more. To those who saw vital force as somehow related to the electrical nature of the nervous impulse, the worry was that there was, in the words of Charles Rosenberg, a "necessarily limited quantity of vital energy and . . . innumerable possibilities for energy loss from within the closed system that was the human organism. . . . A fixed quantity of nervous force, a hereditary endowment assumed to be electrical in nature, filled and coursed through the channel that was the nervous system. . . . An adequate physiological response meant equilibrium and health, an inadequate one instability and thus disease."[1] What was correct on an individual level was true on a cultural level as well. Society could not progress without a careful allocation of its resources. There were not enough good manners, good will, desirable acquaintances, high wages, political honesty to go around. The assumption of scarcity, fundamental to this reasoning, was a concept which persisted into the twentieth century, elaborated by Havelock Ellis and Sigmund Freud as the theory of sublimation: that some appetites need be subordinated to others was a characteristic of civilization.[2]

Given this limitation of all resources, but especially energy, it was essential not to fritter one's very life away in meaningless or destructive behavior or thoughts. Only an ordered existence made sense, one in which the individual's marshaled resources were carefully expended rather than prodigally squandered. If late Victorian Americans were sure about the appropriateness, even the morality, of order, they were uncertain as to its ultimate sources, and hence as to the means by which to instruct the maintenance of order. Fastidious in drawing distinctions between the civilized and the savage, they were nevertheless ambivalent about both civilization and noncivilized states. Where was true order to be found and if it could indeed be found, how did it manifest itself in human behavior? How did individuals know the proper way to behave, and did this knowledge itself ensure their proper conduct or were sanctions necessary to enjoin them to act in their own—and society's—best interests?

These were concerns which the social arrangements of late nineteenth-century America certainly exacerbated. Without either the controls of a small, face-to-face society, or of anything remotely approaching a totalitarian state, it was crucial to encourage individuals to become as self-governing as possible. This was a difficult task to undertake when people's experiences and degrees of autonomy and power differed so widely, and when the sources of ideological and structural authority were so much in question. Advisors rejected the dichotomous model of either giving oneself up to uncontrolled impulses or completely squelching them. Obviously, they did not want to create libertines; nor did they wish to produce automatons: instead they wished to engender individuals who were as self-determining, comfortably functioning, and socially responsible as possible, given the limited human resources and uncertain social context within which they felt they were operating. Rather than oppressing the appetites and passions, they wished to inculcate the self-ordered, self-repressed expression of them.

Self-repressed expression is not necessarily a contradiction in terms. Constraint, suppression, or oppression continually imposed and reinforced from without were not at the core of most advice literature. Self-control, self-repression (which is repression in the technical Freudian sense), and sublimation were central to this as to so many ideological elements of late nineteenth-century liberal, capitalist America. The essential questions with which to approach this ideology are: What was each person expected to repress and sublimate? What was each person expected to express? By what means was the balance of control and expression to be achieved? As Dr. Henry Maudsley, the English neurologist and popularizer of medical-psychological theories, explained to his wide American readership: "It is not by eradication but by wise direction of the egoistic passions, not by annihilation but by utilization of them that progress in social

77

culture takes place." Maudsley denounced oppressive Christian theologians, who, he believed, sought to condemn all the powers of instinctual life. "One can only wonder at the absurdly unpractical way in which theologians have declaimed against them, as though it were a good man's first duty to root them clean out of his nature, and as though it were their earnest aim to have a chastity of impotence, a morality of emasculation."[3]

Although he was writing about all the drives, Maudsley chose sexual metaphors, more specifically metaphors of male castration anxiety, to vent his anger toward those whom he considered to be the oppressors. Despite their general concerns with what was to be self-repressed and what expressed, the advisors wrote more about sexual drives than about the control of hunger, aggression, or any other drives they saw as vital to life. A central human function in itself, sexuality also exemplified both the private area of behavior which needed self-policing and appropriate expression, and the relationship between the personal and the social spheres. The problems of power relationships between the sexes and classes, the thin line between individualism and antisocial behavior in all spheres, anxiety about deploying resources —all bedeviled social as well as personal relationships. Sexuality was a subject, in this sense a political subject, to which the advisors had apparently given much thought, seeing in its proper use a model for the rest of a well-lived life. One can perceive in their advice their struggle to make sense of the expression of this appetite.[4] Sexuality was an especially perplexing phenomenon in these years. Changes in the functions of sexuality when combined with the difficulties of finding the appropriate modes of impulse control made sexual behavior, responsibilities, beliefs, and fantasies all potent metaphors for the conduct of life. Baffled and troubled, most advisors entered the ongoing discussion in a pessimistic frame of mind. They saw in their contemporaries' lives much evidence of antisocial sexual behavior and sexual dysfunction which caused torment in individual lives and disruption in society.

Their concerns often fluctuated from the superficial to the

profound, from anxiety over the frequency of sexual intercourse to worry that separating sexuality from reproduction would cause social chaos. In the welter of warnings, suggestions, and explanations, a number of preoccupations emerge. Especially disturbing to many advisors was the reduced fertility rate of American women. This had been a source of comment in popular magazines even before 1870. As we have pointed out in chapter 1, by 1880, the United States had a lower ratio of children to women of childbearing age than did any Western European nation save France. This change reverberated on many levels. Since no advisors indicated that marriage itself was becoming more unusual, they concluded that the uses made of marriage were changing, as indeed they probably were, given the gradual loss of independent production from the household, the increased tendency for the husband to be a full-time wage earner, the wife to take on economic, social, and psychological functions quite apart from the husband's, and for children to be in school. For a variety of reasons, both in country and in city, the need for and desire to have large families was not always apparent, nor was the economic nature of marriage. Toward what ends, then, was the conjugal relationship directed? A committee reporting in 1868 to the General Assembly of the Presbyterian church, which endorsed its findings, thought it knew the answer: "With great pain we are constrained to admit the increasing prevalence in many parts of our country, of unscriptural views of the marriage relation." As reasons for this unfortunate phenomenon, it pointed to the "growing devotion to fashion and luxury" of the age and to "the idea which practically obtains to so great an extent, that pleasure, instead of the glory of God and the enjoyment of His favor, is the great object of life."[5] If the advisors sensed that sex was being employed increasingly not only by the young and unattached, but also by husbands and wives for purposes other than procreation, then the restraints on sexual behavior built into procreative sex would be less meaningful than they once had been. Sexuality unleashed from reproduction was potentially sexuality granted infinite play. This was an unacceptable prospect to those who felt that "love must submit to discipline, to order," and to feminists who worried that in a society of inequality between the sexes, women could only lose an important source of economic support, indeed of leverage in conjugal relations, if the marriage relation were no different than legalized prostitution.[6]

The dilemmas provoked by the separation of sexuality from procreation found their expression partly in the debates and struggles over contraception and abortion. Abortion, according to James C. Mohr, "entered the mainstream of American life during the middle decades of the nineteenth century." By this, he means that its use spread temporarily from the "unmarried and socially desperate" who had always used it to the "white, Protestant native-born wives of middle and upper-class standing" who began using it as a means of family limitation without damaging "irreparably [their] social standing."[7] Physicians who wrote about "criminal abortion" fumed that women, cool as cucumbers, came into their offices demanding abortions, expressing "real or pretended surprise that anyone should deem the act improper—much more guilty." These "educated, refined, and fashionable women" were not altogether unwilling to bear children—physicians acknowledged them to be possessed of "an ardent and self-denying affection to the children who already constitute the family"—but after a given number of offspring, they were "perfectly indifferent respecting the fetus in utero."[8]

The late nineteenth-century proliferation of contraceptive devices, from rubber condoms to syringes for douching, from pessaries for "uterus support" to patent medicines, from sponges to folk recipes, led some physicians to fulminate publicly against the physically injurious effects of every known technique. Others, medical and lay people alike, declared their hostility to contraceptive techniques as frauds which would debase the quality of the moral relation between husband and wife, would license promiscuity, and would lead to marital breakdown. "I am old-fashioned enough," William Goodell told his medical students in 1879, "to believe that pregnancy is a necessary condition to healthful and happy marriages, and further that coition is innocuous only when complete in both husband and wife, and when the germinal fluid bathes her reproductive organs."[9]

Some physicians, troubled by widespread criminal abortion and by the prospect of losing their leadership role on this issue to others, explored the perimeters of justifiable birth control. Occasionally, by explicitly and publicly advocating specific contraceptives, physicians would risk prosecution under the 1873 Comstock Law, which made dissemination of contraceptive information and devices illegal. Many doctors were torn: on the one hand, they felt that sex could not and should not be confined to propagative purposes, and on the other hand, they could not bring themselves to open the Pandora's box of birth control. "Until a very recent period, I thought that a physician was not justified in giving any other advice [than continence]," a Wisconsin doctor confessed to his colleagues in 1888, "but now I am looking for more light on the subject."[10] By 1890, there were doctors who suggested in print that wholesale condemnation of contraception on moral grounds was a disservice.

The decline in fertility as achieved deliberately by middle-class women's use of abortion and contraceptives produced anxiety on multiple levels. As in other areas of their lives, middle-class Americans were here, too, in the realm of sexuality, producing less that could be seen and evaluated; the literature reveals advisors' efforts to comprehend an absence which could not be ignored. Andrew Nebinger's complaint about criminal abortion in 1870 was that it resulted in the "non-production of offspring on the part of the American," while twenty years later a less worried Dr. Davendorf wanted to eliminate the evasive moralism, and get down to the real issues: he himself thought it "for the good of humanity to limit the number of children."[11] The general concern over production was by the end of the century honed to a finer edge; it was the non-Anglo-Saxons who were doing the producing. The fear of people like Nathan Allen that the mental work of those possessing the highest state of "refinement, culture and civilization" resulted in a withdrawal of nutrition to the reproductive organs, was heightened by the realization that those people were actually helping along the degenerative process by voluntarily restricting their offspring.[12] The physicians who responded to Andrew Nebinger's questionnaire on abortion in 1870 informed him that criminal abortion was more common in the better classes of society than among the poor, and among Protestants than among Catholics or Jews.[13] As the anonymous author of *The Truth About Love* put it, "When the race sets about enjoying itself, without any reference to offspring, then destruction and death will follow." This author's grim solution was that "the individual must find his satisfaction in subordinating self to race."[14]

The nagging feeling that contraception and abortion meant sex without anything to show for it, work without a product, may serve as well as a partial explanation for the increased Victorian antipathy to masturbation. Masturbation certainly involved a substantial expenditure of energy without any gains that the advisors could see. The masturbator was the self-made man par excellence, and as such he may have served as the focus of some of the ambivalences Americans felt for the idealization of the individual at the expense of ties and obligations to others. A self-absorbed, possessed, selfish person who did not need nor heed others, the masturbator ultimately had nothing left over for anyone else. William Hammond observed of the chronic male masturbator that "he no longer desires intercourse," and worried further that "such persons . . . become often true misogynists."[15] Perhaps, then, masturbation was also a sign that the separate spheres of men and women were in danger of becoming so distinct that no links would remain between the two sexes.

Women's behavior often lent support to the supposition that they were insufficiently assiduous in fulfilling their responsibilities to the other sex. Nancy F. Cott argues that nineteenth-century women often used passive resistance, or passionlessness. Hugh Hodge's complaint was that women were unwilling to pay the piper: "Every obstetrician can bear testimony to the great difficulty of inducing our wayward patients to forego gratifications, to practice certain self-denials."[16] This suggests yet another nerve irritated by the changes in fertility patterns and concomitant altered social relationships. The insubordination of American women, demonstrated in many facets of nineteenth-century life, found expression in the sexual sphere, too, and was debated among the advisors. Women's refusal to honor their marriage relation when it did not please them, to carry on the reproduction which traditionally had been expected of them, to take their doctor's advice on these subjects, and, in general, to accept their lot in life provoked many advisors. To what degree physicians retaliated with sadistic and punitive treatment of their female patients is not clear from the advice literature. Advisors were more likely to rail against the immorality of criminal abortion or contraceptives and then to blunt the implications of their reproaches by concluding that women's actions were owing to their ignorance of the moral or physiological facts. Providing these facts to women created a legitimate role for late nineteenth-century advisors, while denouncing women as immoral limited sales.[17]

The same evidence on at least one of these grounds—refusal to honor the marriage relation—received another interpretation by some advisors in concert with feminists and free lovers. Although they frequently opposed contraception and abortion, these groups saw as valid women's refusal to submit unwillingly to their husbands' sexual demands. To them, the negative results of separating sex from procreation were that the husbands, lacking adequate guidelines for their behavior, took advantage of "the traditionally assertive force of men."[18] In a period in which women were decidedly chafing against their subordinate position in the family and were exploring means of redressing the balance of authority in marriage to permit their own development as individuals, giving up the struggle to control sexual expression in marriage was unthinkable for feminists and for many nonfeminist women as well. Not all writers of this persuasion carried their advocacy of women's insubordination to the same degree, of course. Horatio Storer, an orthodox physician and pioneer warrior against abortion, demanded only that "one simple rule . . . be observed, that the husband compel his wife to do nothing she herself does not freely assent to."[19]

Beyond this, feminists and free lovers were united in their insistence that women be the ones to determine when and if they should get pregnant; this is the position Linda Gordon has described as *voluntary motherhood*. To complaints that the "best" women were having the fewest children, they retorted that the future of the race depended upon the high quality of children that could be born only to willing mothers. Elizabeth Cady Stanton, who from 1869 to 1880 traveled the lyceum circuit lecturing to mixed audiences on "Home Life" and "Our Girls" and to thousands of eager women on "Marriage and Maternity," urged not only voluntary motherhood, but dissolvable marriage as well. Many marriages, she thought, were devoid of real feeling, were "feeble, indifferent, joyless, discordant unions." Such relationships, contracted out of necessity, accident, or ignorance, could not produce worthy offspring. For women's own sakes and for those of their potential children, she advocated divorce to end unsuccessful unions and urged "enlightened motherhood." Hal Sears writes of nineteenth-century free lovers that "the word 'free' in free love held two meanings for women: the freedom not to surrender their vagina to anybody regardless of their relationship or supposed duty, and the freedom to offer it at will." With the distinction that she disapproved of sexual promiscuity and advocated monogamy for hereditarian reasons, Cady Stanton publicly agreed with this aspect of the free-love advocates' philosophy. That these issues were extremely contentious is illustrated by the fact that Cady Stanton claimed her lectures on marriage and divorce were very well received while conservative feminists objected to her undertaking the subjects at all, and one suffragist remembered 1869 as the year of the free-love panic when "one could hardly speak in the most academic or speculative way of the marriage or divorce question without being accused of free love bias."[20]

The apparently growing insubordination of women in regard to sex was a worrisome reminder that others, too, especially adolescents, acted as they pleased sexually and in other ways as well. Here the focus was on adolescent masturbation which was both troubling in itself and a potential source of trouble for adult reproductive capabilities. The long period between school leaving and marriage in which young people, at this point neither children nor adults, were expected to help the precarious finances of their families through their labor, seems to have been a difficult time for the adult supervisors as well as the adolescent and postadolescent participants.[21] There were so many temptations in modern life to lure young people into behavior both destructive and self-destructive. Parents were often dependent upon the labor of their offspring, but were not in the best position to ensure their good behavior, especially when the young people moved to the cities to find work. Robert Neuman has argued that one of the reasons that adolescent masturbation was so disturbing to parents and physicians was that young people's preoccupation with the activity was both an actual and a symbolic repudiation of adult authority. Offspring would neither study nor work, remaining stubbornly enmeshed in their solitary fantasies, immune to parental strictures on this and other subjects. Parents and physicians noted with disgust the telltale symptoms on once-bright faces: "A besotted, embarrassed, melancholy, and stupid look; loss of all presence of mind; incapability of bearing the gaze of any one . . . indisposition to make any active exertion."[22] Since onanism provided a kind of microcosm of the temptations open to humans which could and should be overcome, it was the responsibility of all parents to give proper instruction to their children while their minds and bodies were still being formed. Controlling this dangerous nonproductive urge would be one of the best grounds for character training, for the establishment of good personal and social habits. In regard to their male offspring, parents were urged to "teach him that his early inclination to seek such pleasure is one of his opportunities to test and strengthen his character; that the grade of his manhood is established by the amount he can overcome, and that his value in the world depends much on the question as to whether he will rule his body or his body him."[23] Even the language here betrays the anxiety over authority and the tendency to insubordination.

Furthermore, masturbation in the early years, because of the dangers in premature uses of organs, was often believed to be one cause of impotence in adult males. "Most of the cases of impotence which medical men have to treat," William Hammond wrote in *Sexual Impotence in the Male,* "are the result of excessive and premature indulgence in masturbation rather than in sexual intercourse." "When they marry, [masturbators] find that sexual intercourse is far from satisfying their desire, and moreover, that it is less excitant of the genesic feeling than the habit in which they have indulged. They avoid it, therefore, and practice in secret the vice to which they are devoted."[24] Hence masturbation, in addition to hindering the work of young people, would cripple their reproductive capabilities as adults.

Judging from the amount written about it, and the attention focused on it, sexuality and its expressions bore far more than their deserved share of the concern over changes in people's lives. In many instances, individuals and groups responded to unease by attempting to regularize and limit sexual expression in order to stop changes that were already well under way. Passage of the Comstock Act and the various state anticontraceptive laws bespoke both what Daniel Scott Smith calls "an objective increase in 'deviant' behavior" and a desperate awareness that self-repression was not working as it presumably had in earlier, more innocent times. The arrest and prosecutions of more than forty medical entrepreneurs and physicians during the 1870s for performing abortions, and the convictions of more than twenty of them, did not stem the tide of declining fertility, changing marriages, restless women, and wayward adolescents.[25] Neither did the laws achieve the feat of banishing threatening practices through silence; sex radicals added the free expression of ideas to their campaign for the appropriate expression of their feelings, and doctors, in denouncing all available forms of birth control, save abstinence, as injurious, described in some detail the offending devices and techniques.[26]

The prohibitionist efforts to control anxiety by severely limiting expression, while illustrative of the use of sex as the focus of concerns about the balance between expression and sublimation, do not convey the entire picture, however. There were many participants in the public forum who were no less troubled by the same issues, whose conclusions and recommendations were not to close off discussion or to forbid by law a wide range of behavior, but to provide guidelines for the appropriate expression of the sexual and other appetites. Finding themselves in the midst of change, they pondered the sources of instinctive behavior and participated in the emergence of a revised sexual ideology to explain and influence this behavior.

6

The Rule of
Moderation in
Sexual Ideology

Henry Maudsley's general warning that "it is not by eradication but by wise direction of egoistic passions, not by annihilation, but by utilization of them, that progress in social culture takes place," captures the tone of many of the advice writers on sexuality.[1] They could see compelling arguments for both expression and self-restraint. How to benefit from the dynamism of one without losing the predictability and orderliness of the other was the essential dilemma, analogous perhaps to the mixture of exhilaration and fear provoked by the unruly industrial capitalism of the nineteenth century. There were those like Elizabeth Blackwell, one of the first American-trained women physicians, who sometimes focused on the deployment of scarce resources: "The healthy limitation of sexual secretion in men sets free a vast store of nervous force for employment in intellectual and practical pursuits. . . . Even in strong adult life there is great loss of social power through the squanderings of adult energy."[2] Other writers, like R. V. Pierce, made clear the fit between liberal democracy and self-repression: "In all cultures there must be self-control, and the practice of self-denial at the command of love and justice is always a virtue. Self-government is the polity of our people, and we point with pride and laudable exaltation to our political maxims, laws and free institutions. The family is the prototype of society. If self-restraint be practiced in the marital relation, then the principle of self-control will carry health, strength, and morality into all parts of the commonwealth."[3]

In an era in which excess seemed to characterize so much of American economic and political life, Pierce saw social order and the clearly implied possibility of disorder both deriving from the individual. The earlier nineteenth-century notion that individual perfection would bring social redemption had by no means disappeared even though the possibility being offered here was less of perfection than of stability.

On the other hand, advisors explicitly stated that the moderate expression of sexual appetites was essential to good health and happiness. The same advisor who saw self-control as emanating from the individual was also certain, as were many authors, that passion was an essential part of the human character. "The creator has endowed men and women with passions, the suppression of which leads to pain, their gratification to pleasure, their satiety to disgust." Some advisors warned that unfulfilled physiological functions would lead to illness. "As sex is a natural and most powerful human force, there is risk of injury in permanently stifling it," wrote one doctor who was urging young people to marry in their twenties while they were at the height of their vigor. At the same time, a minister counseled young men, "Though a good sexual endowment prove a curse when uncontrolled, yet it was given to us for our own good. Take it away, and you rob us of almost everything. . . . Sexuality is the absolute foundation of manhood and womanhood."[4] In a book titled *Excessive Venery,* another writer ascribed to continence many of the same diseases often blamed on overindulgence: impotence, spermatorrhea, satyriasis in men; and nymphomania and hysteria in women. The belief that intemperance at either end of the spectrum would yield similar ill effects is illustrated further by the admonition of one physician that "the reports of lunatic asylums show that unbridled sexual indulgence is a factor in producing mental disorders, and [that] it is equally certain that undue restraint of a natural and necessary exercise of the sexual instinct is likewise a prominent cause of insanity."[5]

Not simply sexual expression, but sexual pleasure of a specifically genital variety, was, to many advisors, necessary to avoid physiological and emotional disorders on the part of husband and wife. Speaking to both sexes, one writer maintained categorically that "any sexual embrace not attended with sexual orgasm, is very detrimental, and causes diseases,"[6] while another author, refuting the popular notion that "a certain degree of pleasurable feeling, at the crisis of the copulative act, constituting the sexual orgasm is essential to impregnation," nevertheless insisted that "the sexual orgasm on the part of the female is just as normal as on the part of the male."[7] To Henry G. Hanchett, the health of a marriage as well as that of the participants was dependent upon the exchange of sexual pleasure; a marriage without the enthusiastic sexual participation of the wife as well as of the husband was bound to fail. As a woman neglecting to respond to her husband's sexual desires would lose his affection, it was her compelling "duty to her husband, her children and herself, to heartily enjoy with her husband sexual intercourse, and to keep herself in such condition that she may enjoy it."[8] Here, orgasm, as opposed to frigidity, became an obligatory social goal for the self-disciplined woman. This formulation well illustrates what we mean by self-repressed expression. Not only was Hanchett implicitly criticizing those who thought sex should play but a very limited role in marriage, and those who accepted female frigidity as normal, he was also countering feminist efforts to release wives from sexual "duties" by at once threatening them with the loss of their livelihood if they resisted, and offering them pleasure in exchange for acceptance.

93

Hanchett's express concern for the health of marriages also illustrates an effort on the part of many advisors to formulate a legitimate reason for the expression of marital sexuality. Implicitly acknowledging that the primary *raison d'être* of middle-class marriages was no longer the production of a large number of offspring, these writers justified sexual expression in terms of the bonding effect it had upon marriage partners and the reward it offered for other sacrifices. Horatio Storer, who launched his career as an antiabortionist, at the same time acknowledged that the "pleasures of venery . . . restrained within bonds as to frequency . . . serve to add a charm to life, and to give fresh courage for enduring all its vicissitudes." George L. Austin, whose *Perils of American Women* contains one of the rare physiological descriptions of sexual intercourse, held a more exalted view of "the purpose of coition," which was "to bring about unification in the nature of the couple, to facilitate the assimilation of the physical and moral qualities of both." Austin believed that the husband's semen fecundated the entire woman, giving her many qualities of character not possessed before marriage, while Elizabeth Blackwell maintained that "marriage [was sex's] true method of expression and education."[9] Thus by the late nineteenth century many advisors were stressing the pleasure-giving functions of heterosexual sex, rightly understood, beyond the merely procreative function. However, these defenders of qualified sexual pleasure did not prescribe that fulfillment in and of itself—that is, pleasure was to be fostered to serve a primarily nonsexual, even conservative, purpose, the enrichment and stabilization of the family. Tying sexual pleasure solely to the marital relationship and making it serve that relationship would be one means of grasping at stability at a time of transition. These advisors were seeking to turn behavior which others saw as a threat to the family into a reinforcement of a partly redefined marital relationship.

Nevertheless, not all advisors were willing to acknowledge an enriched marriage as a sufficient justification for sexual expression. Some saw as inadequate the self-imposed limitations on intimate behavior that would operate from this emphasis. To these advisors, purists that they were, sexuality for reproduction alone was the only feasible way of attaining the right balance between repression and expression. In their construction, sexual pleasure was an entirely incidental side effect of the reproductive act; unrelated to possible procreation, incontinence was wrong. "The pleasure attached to this function is simply to insure reproduction and nothing more," one purist asserted. "The gratification of this passion, or indeed of any other, beyond its legitimate end is an undoubted violation of natural law, as may be determined by the light of nature, and by the resulting moral and physical evils."[10] Others (a distinct minority) extended their argument further to bolster their fight against lasciviousness. "While any mere sensual indulgence is unworthy and degrading, let it be understood that continence is wholesome and honorable." Where an advisor justifying sexual expression within marriage saw marriage thus defined as the supreme test of human self-control, this writer viewed continence as the epitome of self-control over the lurking passions.[11]

These examples illustrate in part the range of opinion on the appropriate expression of sexuality. At one end of the spectrum were those of an ascetic frame of mind who were wary of the demoralizing and unhealthy effects of distorted appetites, and those who wished to cleanse society through purified intimate relations between the sexes, especially in individuals' roles as parents, passing on to their children the benefits of a carefully preserved heredity. As sexual purists, or evangelicals, as Charles Rosenberg and Philip Greven call them, they contributed openly to the discussion on appropriate sexual behavior.[12] In the middle of the spectrum were the majority of the advisors who were searching for somewhat more flexible, balancing principles of behavior with which individuals and their society could feel as comfortable as possible given the goal of stable, monogamous, heterosexual marriage. At the other end of the spectrum were those whose ideal was gluttony of all the senses, who, in sexual terms, dreamed of pornotopia. Since the market for their writings was more specialized and their offerings less readily available, we are not dealing with them here, although in a perverse way they were commentators on more widely shared values.

In their efforts to balance control with correct expression, not just of sexuality but of all the appetites, the mainstream advisors, inevitably one supposes, settled upon the concept of moderation to describe the balancing principle they were seeking. Moderation was not something they sought to impose artificially, but was presumed organic to the workings of nature. In their own eyes, the sexual advisors, like all the instructors we have been discussing, were not merely applying negative moral strictures to behavior, but were helping their readers function better by uncovering the physiological laws which they assumed underlay the universe. Even the purpose of human sexual intercourse was the subject of such laws: "This is a question that will be, must be, and should be investigated, for, whatever is the law established in the constitution of human beings, it is for their highest good to understand and obey it. Causes and consequences are as unalterably related in the organic as in the inorganic world. . . . With Nature all is law—absolute, invariable, irreversible, eternal."[13] The advisors concluded that moderation was a principle inherent in nature: "It is a physiological fact that the moderate use of any function contributes to health, longevity, and enjoyment, while excessive indulgence is punished with physical ills."[14]

As self-evident as this principle was meant to be, it was not possible for the instructors to reach consensus on its application. If moderation was a rule that could be of help in providing day-to-day guidelines for sexual behavior, it could not tell the anxious reader where that behavior originated, and without knowing that, how could one decide which of competing claims to moderation was correct? For instance, if sex were perceived as the inheritance from the older, baser parts of human nature, then it might be necessary to keep this animal part well in check lest it extend its domain over the more evolved portions of human nature. Eliza B. Lyman, a sexual purist, reasoned that "man's physical functions are as purely animal as those of his lower kin, and the more implicitly he obeys the natural laws governing the animal functions, the more robust and symmetrical he will become." She gave lip service to the importance of both natures, higher and animal: "Each department has its own work and one is just as sacred as the other." However, she concluded that "man has been endowed with reason to guide him and keep him above the brute. The angel nature was placed uppermost to hold in check the animal passions. The greatest wrong from which Humanity suffers today comes through an abuse of the sexual nature."[15]

Lyman urged the use of reason as a guide to sexual behavior. Elizabeth Blackwell had a reading of sexual problems more subtle than a mind/body split. She saw sex as a neutral, physical act which was vulnerable to the influence of that very mind which separated humans from animals. "It is this mental sentiment peculiar to human sex which is capable of a two-fold development. It may grow into a noble sympathy, self-sacrifice, reverence, and joy, which enlarge and intensify the nature through the gradual expansion of the inborn moral elements of sex." The mind, properly developed and used, would bring out the best in sex. One could not absolve oneself of responsibility by claiming that one's animal nature got the best of oneself. The body was, after all, the servant of the mind. On the other hand, if one were lax about cultivating good mental habits, permitting dissolute thoughts, then sexual expression would show the influence of this fevered imagination. Such abuse of the sexual function was not to be found in the simpler animal world. "It is the degradation of this mental power when running riot in unchecked licence that converts men and women into selfish and cruel devils— monsters quite without parallel in the brute creation."[16]

Emphasizing the development of the mind while distrusting the fantasies welling up from what would later be called "the unconscious," Blackwell's perception of the origin of sexual health and disease focused on the interior drama. For other writers the drama was more exterior, taking the form of the corruption of a simple, instinctual act by a complex civilization.

"Modern civilization places us . . . in such an unnatural position," one writer concluded, that sexual behavior is simply "not satisfactorily governed by our own instincts and desires." Social decadence, asserted another writer, had created such a corrupt humanity that natural, instinctual man was simply an irrelevancy. "The lustful cravings of our pampered selves is no more nature than is a call for brandy a natural appetite." Sexual degradation was an acquired characteristic, force-grown in the fetid soil of modern society. "When the passions are stimulated by unnatural habits of living, by impure conversation, thoughts, books and practices; can we say this strength of passion is purely natural and healthy?" Pure-food advocates tended to focus on unnatural and adulterated foods as the culprits here: coffee, tea, alcohol, spicy foods, and, to many, meat fell under the ban. To this list John Cowan added tight lacing, a fashion which others decried for its detrimental effects on women's health. He denounced tight lacing because "the constricting of the waist and abdomen by corsets, girdles and waistbands, prevents the return of the venous blood to the heart, and [he also denounced] the consequent overloading of the sexual organs, and, as a result, of the unnatural excitement of the sexual system."[17] One advisor suggested that the nobel savage who was so in tune with nature handled his sexuality easily, and that sexual obsession grew in modern urban civilization. "Those who live outdoors and have well-balanced constitutions of the old-fashioned sort are not annoyed by sexual desire when they have no opportunities for gratification nor to the same degree as the delicate, finely-organized lads of our cities and of the higher civilization."[18] To those whom Hal Sears has called "sex radicals," civilization was destructive, not so much in the temptations it offered to artificially inflame the passions, but in the arbitrary restrictions it imposed on the natural reason possessed by every individual.

George Beard, the advisor who thought that preoccupation with sex was a side effect of modern urban civilization, presumed, at his most optimistic, that human beings and human society would evolve to a stage in which they were once more in harmony. Pure-food advisors such as John H. Kellogg and Russell T. Trall felt that by living naturally and correctly, humans could immediately reattune themselves with their instincts: "The more nearly the parties live in accordance with physiological habits, especially in the matters of food, clothing and exercise, the more nearly normal will be their sexual inclinations, and the less need they have of subjecting their desires to the restraints or control of reason."[19] Trall suggested that through a stripping away of unnatural habits, one could return to a state of nature where the instincts would be sound and behavior naturally moderate. However, this ideal of the naturally sound individual was not generally shared by the other advisors; they presumed that rational control over the dangerous appetites, whether conceived of as instinctual or as the results of overcivilization, would always be necessary.[20]

Consequently, they felt the need to spell out a sexual hygiene, to detail a framework for moderate sexual expression. While the advisors' guidelines depended upon their assumptions about the origins of sexual behavior and the function of sexuality, most readers, no doubt, culled what they wanted or needed from the specifics they were given, not being able to decide with any finality the ultimate meaning of sex. Few, if any, of the sex guides had an exuberant, self-confident view of sexual expression, and so the reader was given the impression that moderate sexual expression was like a path through a minefield, a risky trek requiring markers both for the danger spots and for the safe areas.

Many advisors felt that one of the chief markers they could provide for their readers to aid them in charting a successful course through their sexual lives was that of suitable frequency of sexual intercourse. This was in keeping with the widespread concern over the limitation of resources and the presumed necessity to direct one's energies where they would best contribute to personal and social progress. Warnings about frequency, most often directed toward males, may also have been one way in which mainstream advisors dealt with the complaints of many feminists and male sexual purists about the unrelenting sexual demands made by insensitive husbands upon their overworked wives.[21] Advice about frequency varied according to the function which advisors assigned to sexuality. John Cowan, a fanatic among purists, argued for the one perfect sex act per well-spaced, wanted child. Although he abhorred sex in any other context than the reproductive, Cowan by no means suggested a tight-lipped, joyless fumbling in the dark. It may have been his advocacy of the one consummate act as a beautiful, special rite which contributed to the endorsement of him by feminist Elizabeth Cady Stanton, who was also an admirer of the poetry of Walt Whitman, as well as a believer in high quality marriage between equals and in wanted children. Cowan advised: "Now the best and only physiological time to generate a new life is in the broad light of a clear, bright day. Light implies health, darkness disease. . . . Keeping their natures as is the bright sun, with not the smallest cloud intervening to darken their joy and happiness [the husband and wife] enter their chamber and in the clear light of day the New Life is conceived and generated—a new soul started into eternity."[22]

Even those who regarded sex as a more continual part of marriage, perhaps even accepting the validity of birth control, felt it necessary to provide guidelines about frequency. Each individual involved should always be aware of his or her physical limitations in order to self-monitor sexual activity. The application of this principle was extended to both sexes, although concern for the male was clearly dominant. Thus the moderate William A. Hammond, who counseled many patients with sexual problems, indicated that guidelines should be chosen on a self-conscious, individual basis. "It is exceedingly difficult to lay down any rule in the matter which will be applicable for all men; indeed, the task would be insuperable, for all men are not alike, and what would be excess for one would be moderation for another." He did feel, however, that he could safely make a few mercantilist generalizations: "Twice a week is certainly excess for the majority of men, and will certainly lead to earlier than normal extinction of the sexual powers. Once a week is more generally applicable. . . . If the individual desires to retain his ability to a green old age, he will not tax it too severely in his youth."[23] Hammond's conclusions were in line with that of most advisors. Edward Bliss Foote generally agreed with such a timetable, but he buttressed his notions as to frequency with an electrochemical explanation. For Foote, the acidic semen was to strike the alkaline vaginal secretions for the proper electrical effect: "Several days, and sometimes weeks, must elapse, after one indulgence, before the secretions of the vagina will become so purely alkaline as to be prepared for another animated combination with the acid of the male."[24] George M. Beard, on the other hand, relied more upon psychological factors in determining the frequency of safe indulgence, stressing that the way sexuality was used determined its consequences. "There is no doubt that excess with a mistress or excess with a public woman is more liable to bring on genital debility than excess in the married—for this psychological reason, that when we visit a mistress, or when we visit a public woman, we go solely, or mainly, at least, for the purpose of sexual gratification; our minds are upon the idea; consequently there is a constant excitation of the sexual function." He compared this scenario with that of married life where "we live constantly with our companion; in such a relation the sexual act is incidental, and therefore less exhausting to the nerves."[25]

Another marker on the path of safe sexual expression besides frequency was periodicity, about which advisors agreed in general although they disagreed on particulars. Since moderate sexual expression was most attainable at certain times in the life cycle, advisors frequently warned their readers about premature or inappropriate sex in the form of childhood masturbation, indulgence during pregnancy or menstruation or post-menopausal copulation—all of which violated the rules of sexual health.

On the whole, these authors presumed that childhood sexuality was abnormal, a learned rather than a natural characteristic. "If raised strictly in accordance with natural law, children would have no sexual notions or feelings before the occurrence of puberty," one sexual purist asserted. However, he continued, this "natural state" was only "rarely seen in modern homes. Not infrequently, evidences of sexual passion are manifested before the child has hardly learned to walk." For him, "incipient vices" were "planted and fostered" by the parents in the home itself.[26] For other writers, nursemaids or school chums were the culprits; but in any event, childhood sexuality could be developed to pathological proportions by corrupt associations and practices.

The advisors felt that there were sound physiological reasons to abhor precocious sexuality. As Hammond warned, "It is a law of the organism that any function which is over-exerted before the organs producing it are fully matured is certain to lead to the derangement or even extinction of that function." Like the advice over the frequency of sexual expression, the concern with periodicity was in part grounded in the model of limited human resources. "A child whose brain is overtaxed by studies, which are in advance of those suitable for an immature brain, runs serious risks of becoming epileptic or imbecile. Another, who is set to the performance of physical work of too severe a character, is arrested in its growth, and becomes puny and feeble; and it is equally certain that a like result, so far as regards the generative system, will follow on a too early excitation of the sexual organs."[27]

This principle extended right through adolescence, which was the period of maximum growth when all energies were to be reserved rather than dissipated. Only terrible results would follow from breaking down the body when it should be abuilding. One instructor detailed the dangers: "To use before the time, the pleasures of love, is to arrest its growth, to make a delicate complexion, emaciated muscles, feeble organs, poor blood. Moreover, in proportion as there is a hereditary or acquired predisposition to any constitutional disease, a too early conjugal association tends to awaken it,—to make it break forth with violence."[28] This was yet another reason why concern about masturbation was so strong.

The cyclical character of women's reproductive functions demanded a further set of moderating principles on the basis of periodicity. Suggested proscription of sexual intercourse during menstruation, justified on both hygienic and moral grounds, met almost total approval by late nineteenth-century advisors; less unanimous, however, was the censorship of intercourse during pregnancy and after menopause. George L. Austin ascribed morning sickness and miscarriage to sexual relations during the early months of pregnancy. He further argued that since animals abstained from intercourse during pregnancy, asking for similar abstinence on the part of husbands was asking for very little. However, he also observed that most physicians were not concerned with this question and that it appeared that the popular vote was on the side of indulgence. John Cowan predictably and emphatically insisted that the lust accompanying intercourse would damage the foetus itself. "Do not, I pray you, O parents, do this unclean thing. Do not taint your clean bodies, do not foul your pure souls with the lustful parts of your natures, while a new body is being developed, a new soul being organized." Another advisor, on the other side of the argument, was fearful that "ungratified desires, where so great as to gain control of the mind, [were] liable to mark the foetus with an insatiable appetite." Therefore, rather than urging abstinence during pregnancy, he counseled moderation under the belief that "the moderate gratification of any appetite, when consistent with reason, is better than absolute denial."[29]

A few authors assumed that once a woman reached menopause, both her sexual desire and her attractiveness would cease, and would be supplanted by the compensatory virtue of wisdom and the regard of universal esteem: "The body itself does not long delay entering into decrepitude, and soon we see the woman —once so favored by nature when she was charged with the duty of reproducing the species—degraded to the level of a being who has no further duty to perform in the world. However, her family and society recompense her for the loss of her physical charms, by surrounding her with respect and heart-felt care, which are in remuneration for services which she has rendered to one and

another in the past."[30] This was a strictly functionalist argument
about female sexuality; pleasure was scarcely the central end of
sex. Yet, to many it was obvious that sometimes sexual desires
persisted or even increased as a woman passed the age of reproduction. Increased passion where physiological law decreed
cessation to some indicated abnormality and even disease.
The homeopathic physician Prudence B. Saur warned that
menopausal sexuality "should always be looked upon with serious apprehension for it is against nature, and may be the indication of some grave disease. There is no doubt but that sexual
gratification at this time is a very common cause of intensifying
all the numerous inconveniences and ailments which are attend-
ant upon this period." Where Saur advised continence as "not
only recommended but . . . enjoined as one of the most essential
hygienic measures by which a safe and rapid transit through this
period of sexual decline may be insured," others urged temperance instead.[31] Austin, who, it will be remembered, linked morning sickness and miscarriage to sex during pregnancy, explicitly
rejected the view that sexual desire during menopause was pathological. To him, "susceptibility to pleasure" in women past child-
bearing age was normal, and was proof that sexual intercourse
served more than reproductive functions.[32]

Honoring his wife's passage into a postsexual phase, the
decent husband's sex life would be well constrained after middle
age, according to those advisors who felt that moderate sexual
expression would be difficult once the possibilities of procreation
disappeared. In addition, the man's own powers and desires
should be decreasing by this point in his life. In a spirit no more
generous than he displayed toward women's postreproductive
sexuality, Augustus K. Gardner noted that if old men marry
young women, "Nature knows how in such a case to punish
cruelly any infraction of her laws." George H. Napheys urged the
male reader to discipline himself into the role of wise elder lest
he slip into becoming a dirty old man: "He should, as years
progress, steadily wean himself more and more from the control
of desire, and fix his thoughts on those philanthropic and un-

selfish projects which add beauty to age, and are the crown to gray hairs. What more nauseous and repulsive object is there," shuddered Napheys, "than a libidinous and worn-out old man heating his diseased imagination with dreams and images which his chilled and impotent body can no longer carry into effect?"[33] Yet it must be noted that five pages after this admonition Napheys suggested that continued virility was an aid to the postponement of aging!

A final marker on the path of sexual moderation was appropriate sociability, that is, sex taking place between heterosexual, married couples. Premarital, extramarital, homosexual, and autoerotic and other forms of "perverted" sexuality all presented danger signals. George M. Beard, for example, asserted that sex with a mistress or a prostitute, because of the single-mindedness of such relationships, was far more debilitating than married sex in which sexuality was part of a greater range of emotions and activities.

The primary focus for concerns over appropriate sexual sociability was masturbation, which, as Vern L. Bullough and Martha Voght have argued, was something of a code word for a wider and more diffuse range of sexual deviations including homosexuality. Many advisors agonized over the potential for mental debauchery: unlike normal heterosexual union in which the presence of the partner provided sexual stimulus, they feared that masturbation, especially for the male, provoked ceaselessly escalating erotic fantasies on the part of the onanist so that he could achieve the necessary excitation. The advisors worried about the antisocial and uncontrolled quality of these fantasies. Not only would they make the masturbator more vulnerable to a lascivious life, they might also make the normal stimulation of heterosexual activity inadequate for the male to accomplish the sexual act. In describing the chronic adult male masturbator, Hammond observed that "he is, in fact, impotent to woman; he no longer desires intercourse but abandons himself to his fatal habit, knowing the almost limitless resources of his imagination in providing excitations to his desires. Such persons shun the

105

society of women, become often true misogynists, and suffer an entire extinction of the sexual feeling."[34] Hammond ascribed the same dangers to female masturbation, but for most writers, the danger for the female masturbator lay in the opposite direction, in the realm of heightening her vulnerability to the lures of premarital and extramarital sex. "Let this be clearly understood that any indulgence whatever in these evil courses is attended with bad effects, especially because they create impure desires and thoughts which will prepare the girl to be a willing victim to the acts of profligacy."[35] Indeed, these converse admonitions hint that even as late as the end of the nineteenth century, there remained remnants of the earlier belief that women were sexually insatiable. For both sexes, one bad habit engrained in the psyche would lead to a train of others successively more horrid.

Moderation was thus believed to be the royal road to good sexuality as it was to good health in general. Sexual moderation meant not total denial, but self-controlled expression in a most dangerous sector of life, whether the dangers were due to natural disorders or to civilized decay. The same force was potentially both positive and destructive depending upon its use. Sex would function properly if emplaced within marriage, employed with moderate frequency and at the appropriate periods of life, and if it were a social (that is, linking male and female) rather than a selfish act.

Just as in other areas of advice concerning behavior, the emphasis was now on attaining balance more than on achieving perfection, a shift in emphasis from earlier reform beliefs. Even to attain mere moderation was a struggle. While adumbrating the characteristics of good sex, advisors also recognized and described the numerous difficulties standing in its way. The impediments to moderate sexuality loomed ominously large. Biological barriers overlapped with those created by civilization. Natural bodily fragility and limited supplies of energy carried dangers all too often matched by improper socialization. It must be emphasized, however, that this was another area in which advisors disagreed, at least over degree, if not over general principles, and hence gave conflicting signals. Much advice literature gives the impression that not merely was the pool of energy shallow, but the human container of that energy was eggshell thin. It is impossible to know what caused what, but the belief in human vulnerability as opposed to resilience was surely related to fears of imminent chaos in the body politic. Fear of loss was at least as strong as hopes for eventual sufficiency here, as in all health matters.

In the sexual sphere the evident precariousness of function led to such warnings as: "Love does not transmit vitality except at the expense of him who gives it." Where this advisor was categorical in his admonition, others saw variations in the degree of resilience from one person to the next, and thus made their warnings more conditional: "The sexual organs will stand an immense amount of improper usage in the cases of some men; in others however, their power of resistance is much less; and in all, if the excess be continued there is danger that a condition of permanent impotence will be reached." Given this lack of resiliency, it was possible for the individual to minimize loss by exercising care in sexual expression. Excess with a mistress was more debilitating to a man than excess with his wife; expenditure of the vital forces when they occurred would be far less deleterious within connubial confines than if resulting from solitary activity: "During sexual intercourse the expenditure of nerve force is compensated by the magnetism of the partner."[36]

Masturbation often became the focus for fears of fragility and loss, becoming linked as well to otherwise inexplicable forms of nerve disorder and insanity, most particularly epilepsy. For some advisors the nervous effects produced by masturbation paralleled the symptoms of an epileptic seizure; hence masturbation was deduced to be a primary cause of epilepsy. "When we call to mind the immense disturbance of the nervous system consequent upon the development [through masturbation] of the sexual orgasm, the mental vertigo, the muscular convulsion, the cardiac and respiratory excitement, the resemblance which all the phenomena have to those of an epileptic paroxysm into which

they not infrequently pass by an almost imperceptible grada-
tion," William A. Hammond concluded, the dangers of repeated
masturbation were self-evident.[37] Again arguing through parallel
symptoms, many advisors maintained that normal sexual processes in mature life would be undermined by masturbation; the
more premature and excessive the practice, the more severe the
effects. Frigidity, impotence, and spermatorrhea (discharge without orgasm) were the chief results of such excesses.[38]

By no means, however, did all advisors come to such catas-
trophic conclusions about onanism. George M. Beard recognized
these expressions of fear among his contemporaries and sought
to reassure them that masturbation could not be as dire an activity as so many believed, or humankind could not have survived.
"The habit is almost universal. It is indulged in by both sexes. It
is not confined to civilized lands. The semi-barbarous and the
savage are addicted to it," he insisted, pointing out that masturbation was not the result of the social decay of modern civilization. "If it were as prejudicial to the constitution as is currently
believed, the whole earth would be converted into insane asylums, and hospitals for the epileptics. . . . The truth is," he
concluded, "that the genital organs, like the stomach, can bear
and were designed to bear a vast amount of abuse. Had it been
otherwise, the human race would long since have perished from
the earth."[39] As masturbation was so nearly universal, physicians
were often tempted to use it as a lazy (or sometimes cyni-
cal) diagnosis for a variety of ills. One can imagine the doctor
interviewing his patient, learning of his or her history including
masturbation, and stopping right there for his diagnosis. Some
advisors were quite aware of the absurdity of this reliance upon
masturbation as such a general explanation of disease. In his
textbook titled *Diseases of the Urinary and Male Sexual Organs,* the
urologist William T. Belfield commented very shrewdly that if the
patient confessed to have ever masturbated, "the physician is
prone to recognize in this self-pollution that cause of the ill
complained of. Such a course has certainly many advantages: it
affords an easy and tangible diagnosis; it accords with the depen-

dent patient's convictions; and palliates to some extent a possible failure in treatment, by throwing the responsibility upon the guilty patient."[40]

Beard and Belfield were not advocating masturbation, but were simply trying to take the problem out of the hands of the tonic pedlars and fearmongers and to place it in proper perspective. Nevertheless, masturbation was a difficult problem in a society which both delayed the acting out of legitimate sexual expression and feared the more youthful, solitary forms of sexuality. Drawbacks of civilization and flaws in the socialization process were held responsible for many sexual difficulties encountered by adults; masturbation established youthful habits of antisocial and self-injurious behavior which would taint the adult years and weaken the nation.

William Hammond had so many adult male patients with sexual problems that he grouped them in classifications ranging from absence of sexual desire to inability to experience pleasure, and to absence of the power of erection, under which the widespread disorder of partial impotence was subsumed. He noted mental preoccupation, masturbation, perversion of the sexual appetite, business fears, venereal disease, general ill health, lack of self-confidence, and inability to accept sexual desire as legitimate as causes of impotence in males. All of these disorders would affect the man's female sexual partners, especially his wife, and a few of the causes were directly related to perceptions of female sexuality. For instance, one of Hammond's patients, an experienced man of the world who had recently married a "highly educated, intelligent, refined and beautiful woman," was impotent with her in the belief "that it was a profanation for a man like him to subject so beautiful and pure a woman to such an animal relation as sexual intercourse." Hammond assured the anxious husband that "there was no profanation in sexual intercourse, chastely undertaken; that she had sexual organs which were intended for the performance of certain functions," and that he should "lower his estimate of her angelic character and . . . look upon her in the not less worthy light of a woman to be

treated as other women are treated under like circumstances."
Hammond then asked to meet with the wife, whom he found to
be "a very sensible woman, not at all ethereal, but anxious to do
her share towards relieving her husband from his embarrassing
position." Hammond advised her "to be a little more free in her
manner with her husband than she had yet been," leaving the
details "to her own good sense and womanly feeling." The husband returned to Hammond the next day jubilantly exclaiming,
"By Heaven, it reminded me of old times!"[41]

To the degree that sexuality was mutual, women would
suffer from such male limitations as impotence, sexual perversions, and venereal disease, as well as from their own impediments. The limited opportunities for economic independence for
women outside of marriage sometimes made them resentful of
their dependence upon men and of their obligations in the connubial bed. The insensitivity, inexperience, and ineptitude attributed to American men as sexual partners by feminists and
other reformers could not have made these obligations any
sweeter.

Furthermore, there was a discrepancy for women between
the rewards of sexual expression and the price they would have
to pay in terms of unwanted pregnancies, often untreatable
gynecological disorders, and unreliable and often unobtainable
contraceptives. An editorial in an 1888 issue of the *Medical and
Surgical Reporter* indicated that this was "perhaps the most serious
reason why such complaints are made of the excessive indulgence
of the sexual appetite by men. . . . It is not because women have
no corresponding inclination to sexual intercourse in itself which
makes many of them regard it as a burden or a curse, but because
they can rarely rid themselves of the dread of its consequences."[42] Some women still believed that sexual excitement
was necessary to conception and may have consciously or uncon-
sciously dampened their pleasure as a means of contraception.
Advisors often acknowledged the existence of sexual feeling in
women even when they could not bring themselves to advocate

those devices and techniques which would make the expression of womanly passion more carefree.

The authors rarely idealized frigidity among women. Nor did they usually see nonresponsiveness as normal, although neither did they often focus on ways to increase women's sexual pleasure.[43] Here again, William Hammond was an exception. While having little except divorce and a second marriage to suggest to the woman who was married to a man she found repulsive, he was more helpful to the woman who was left behind by her husband's timing. To the too-speedy husband he urged restraint, and to the wife he advocated a prescription for *cannabis* to establish habits of satisfied desire.[44] Some doctors pointed out the physiological and gynecological disorders which accounted for frigidity in women, while many others shared a more general theory: "The social life of woman is such as to impose on her restraints which do not exist, with such full force at least, with the male sex." Alice B. Stockham, who in distributing her book *Tokology* suffered arrest by Anthony Comstock, observed that "we teach the girl repression, the boy expression, not simply by word and book, but the lessons are graven into their very being by all the traditions, prejudices and customs of society." A male advisor bemoaned the fact that women, "having been so persistently and industriously taught that everything connected with the sexual act, or even the sexual organs, is a shame and a disgrace . . . learn after marriage rather slowly and reluctantly what the true estimation, importance, and relations of these organs and act really are."[45]

Although they did not deny the bad effects of biological and social impediments to comfortable sexual expression for women as well as for men, sexual advisors, in advocating moderation, had only relatively weak means by which to palliate or overcome such barriers. If, then, the reservoir of energy were so limited and humans so fragile, moderation, however necessary and useful, was a distinctly limited means to emotional fulfillment. This key to behavior was at best a mode of balance and conservation of energies, rather than a tap into ever-increasing positive force. Although, as we have tried to establish, moderation was not simply a synonym for *suppression* or *oppression,* it tended to underline fears of human inadequacy in the realms of nature and society. Civilization may have required at least some subordination of the sexual drive to other activities, but the advisors did not convey a clear message that the fruits of sublimation were worth having and that civilization brought its own rewards. Some further ideological means was needed to encourage men and women to believe that beyond merely surviving, they could both grow and flourish, that they could have progress and not merely safe stasis. Such a mechanism, apparently, was the assertion of the will.

7

The Primacy
of the Will

I n 1872, William B. Carpenter, possibly the most representative, orthodox, mid nineteenth-century British physiologist, diagramed his model of brain process in *Popular Science Monthly* for his many American readers.[1]

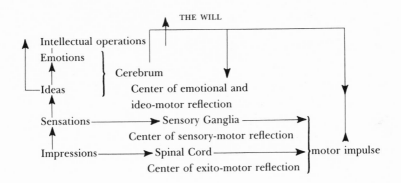

115

Carpenter, although basically a materialist, had here reintroduced supramaterial values by asserting the existence and the primacy of the will. Indeed, it was his intentional linking of moral, psychological, and material categories which made his approach typical.

Although the material model of the brain, which we described in chapter 4, was itself widely accepted, it could not provide an adequate description of the mental processes of human beings; too much was left out, and, most important, there was no place for that sense of dynamism and progress, that individual assertion and improvement so necessary to Victorians, particularly given the stark limitations they attributed to brain capacity and function. Consequently, most medical and popular health writers hedged physiological determinism by incorporating older notions of faculty psychology which included supraphysical states of consciousness such as sensibility, imagination, and judgment as mental characteristics and thus as part of a broader definition of the brain and the mind.[2] Primary among these faculties was the highest human faculty—the will. In his schema, using what he intended to be a materialist framework, Carpenter attempted to find room for an agency of consciousness which would rise above and control automatic and material brain function. In another place, he asserted that "the operations of the Cerebrum are in themselves as automatic as those of other Nerve centers, and that the Volitional control which we exercise over our thoughts, feelings, and actions operates through the selective attention we determinedly bestow upon certain of the impressions made upon the 'Sensorium' out of the entire aggregate brought thither by the nerves of the internal senses."[3] In other words, the will would operate upon the impressions received by the brain, selecting and ranking them before the automatic operations of the cerebrum would take over. Values ascended from the material to the ethereal.

The will, not merely a hedge against physiological determinism, was also a bulwark against the possibility that nature herself and all elements of the human makeup lower than the will were disordered. The will was approached ambivalently: the highest result and best defense of civilization, it was also viewed as an imposed compensation for the loss of good instincts.

It was the will in either event that placed humans above the animals, that enthroned their higher nature above their lower. William James suggested that it was the animal "mind" which condemned it to a lifetime of irresistible instinct and unchangeable routine, while the willfulness of the human mind enabled humans to define their own reality by choice. Even the most thoroughly materialist physiologist, Henry Maudsley, was moved to conclude, "Our appetites and passions prompt or urge their immediate gratification; it is the nobler function of will, enlightened by reason looking before and after, to curb these lower impulses of our nature."[4] If firmly established, the will could control both emotional and physiological workings, thus giving the strengthened individual enormous powers of self-control. "There is no doubt that in those of sound mind," Leonard Corning wrote, "the emotions are capable of being very largely controlled by the will. . . . The emotions, besides being subject to the counteracting influences of the will, are actually capable of being more or less completely suppressed by it."[5] Even in cures for constipation, declared Eliza Lyman, "Above all medical agents in real value is the exercise of the will."[6] R. L. Dugdale in his famous study of the notorious Jukes, went so far as to conclude that in the subworld of degenerates, criminals were better than paupers, distinguished as they were by greater will. "The ideal pauper is the idiotic adult who never could and never will be able to help himself, and may justly be called a living embodiment of death," he maintained scornfully. By contrast (and in retrospect a fine apology for the coexistence of impoverished Americans and robber barons), "the ideal criminal is a courageous man in the prime of life who so skillfully contrives on a large scale that he escapes detection and succeeds in making a community believe him to be honest as he is generous."[7] Other writers, of course, warned against making the one-eyed into kings, insisting that the ends toward which will was applied mattered. Carpenter admonished,

"It must not be forgotten that the Volitional power may be turned to a bad as well as to a good account; and that the value of its results will entirely depend upon the direction in which it is employed."[8] Here, pure will, superman, was not the highest goal; rather, socially accountable, morally conventional willfulness was the general aim.

A central demonstration of the ideological tension between physiological determinism and the insistence upon the primacy of the will was contained in the prevalent definitions of women and judgments of their behavior. This tension also illustrates one of the ways in which women and men were and were not subject to the same standards and guidelines for behavior. The predominant view was that women's biological construction led to immutable behavioral characteristics and roles. Those of the minority dissenting view disputed physiological absolutism and held that malleable social forces essentially determined women's makeup and place. Yet all agreed that women could overcome many of their peculiar limitations through an assertion of the will.

While positing a variety of specific explanations of the biological nature of women, the determinists generally believed that sexual differentiation defined virtually all aspects of women's character. "Solidity and strength are represented in the organization of the male, grace and beauty in that of the female," ran one typical observation. "His broad shoulders represent physical power and the right of domination, while her bosom is the symbol of love and nutrition. . . . Her maternal functions are indicated by greater breadth of hips."[9] Furthermore, in this passage, the social implications of male and female physiological characteristics explained and justified as natural the prevailing organization of American society. Most frequently, biological causation centered on a woman's primary sexual organs. The uterus and ovaries were the governing agents of all a woman's qualities. "By their sympathetic connections, they yield a modifying influence over all the other functions of the system, they mold her character, beautify and perfect her form."[10] Where for the male "the genital apparatus is merely subsidiary, and playing but . . . a very insignificant part in relation to the general [bodily] economy," Horatio R. Storer wrote in his book *Insanity in Women,* "the case is very different [in the female]. Not only is she subject to a host of diseases peculiar to her sex [which] change her natural disposition and character [but] in health, we find her still obedient to a special law."[11]

Sometimes these sexual comparisons centered around aspects of physiology other than the sexual organs, but in every such definition women were distinguished from men, and always to their detriment. For example, S. Weir Mitchell, a noted specialist in women's nervous diseases, argued that breakdown for women was a "far more probable possibility" than for men due to the relative thinness of a woman's blood, an inherent paucity exacerbated by menstruation and childbirth. "As the woman is normally less full-blooded than the man, she is relatively in more danger of becoming more thin-blooded than he."[12] For another writer the essential gender distinction was the smaller "nervous system" in the woman. "In women there is less nervous capacity and vigor, diminished power of control, and a greater readiness to break down under physical and mental strain."[13] In a similar vein, some argued that women's brains were smaller and that there followed "an exact correspondence between brain-substance and intelligence."[14]

Having distinguished women from men physiologically, many authors went on to insist that a special propensity to disease was implicit in women's very natures. As Mitchell wrote a friend: "I think I know something of women; I think I know more about women than most men do. . . . No man knows much about women who has not had under his care a good many sick women. Nothing differentiates the sex so much as sickness."[15] At those periods in their lives in which the sexual function was being established or phased out, women were vulnerable to diseases of all kinds, but especially mental diseases. The "normal" processes of life merged easily into the pathological. In *Perils of American Women,* George L. Austin advised that "at the period of the appearance of menstruation, and at its decadence, special dangers await women, all of them due to their sexual functions." He warned his readers that "on the accession of those feelings of vague uneasiness or positive pain, we frequently find instances in which a dormant tendency to mental disease becomes aroused into action; and acute mania forms one of the risks through which many young women have to pass at the period of puberty."[16] Another hygiene writer maintained that hard-working women, such as farmers' wives, suffered more insanity and other disease because they could not rest during their menstrual periods.[17]

Writers on women's physical nature all agreed that there was a link between a woman's sexual characteristics and hysteria, a disorder to which late nineteenth-century women were indeed prone, but the precise nature of the disease (if indeed it were one) and the causal relationships between emotional and physical states were unclear. For some writers the origins of hysteria were a simple physical matter. Whether a disease of the ovaries, of the uterus, or a tipped womb, disorders of the emotions and the brain would inevitably follow. "Tilt the organ a little forward—introvert it, and immediately the patient forsakes her home, embraces some strange and ultraism—Mormonism, Mesmerism, Fourierism, Socialism, oftener Spiritualism," one medical diagnostician ranted in 1874.[18] For most writers on this subject, norm and aberration, an acceptable level of emotion and morbidly excessive emotionalism, hypersensibility and outright disease, were linked only in vague ways, consequently making the definition of hysteria also hazy. By observing and testing symptoms, the physicians led themselves to believe that hysteria was but the aggravation of woman's natural emotionalism. Thus Mitchell concluded that many of women's unique virtues of character, such as affection, sympathy, and self-denial led directly "to the automatic development of emotion, which, in its excesses and its uncontrolled states, is the parent of much of the nervousness [and hysteria] not due to the enfeeblement of disease."[19]

Some health writers vigorously opposed this specific notion of the genital origins of hysteria as well as the whole wider construct of physiological determinism. It seemed absurd to the regular physician Dr. Ely Van de Warker to place such "undue value . . . to simple ovarian growth and function as a factor in the development of womanly mental and structural peculiarities."[20] The eminent New York physician Stephen Smith felt that many doctors used uterine disease as a catchall explanation for other illnesses a woman might have, thus obviating the need for careful diagnosis while at the same time playing into a woman's worst fears. "Thousands of nervous ladies suffering from some slight and obscure derangements of digestion, or other departure from health, are secretly informed by friends that the womb, that mysterious organ, with its numerous susceptibilities, is liable to an infinite number of strange disorders."[21]

This criticism of physiological determinism was sometimes tied to a broader counterargument that the sickness of American women was caused by the imposition of false and destructive social customs upon women who were by nature healthy. R. T. Trall, for example, regarded women "as the victim[s] rather than the criminal[s]" in their physical weakness. He felt that men first reduced women and then blamed them for their inferiority. Physicians in particular "misled and miseducated" women, thus inducing many "disabilities, follies and infirmities . . . . She has been taught that she is naturally more frail and feeble and prone to disease than man, and that she must be dosed and drugged . . . for the most trivial indispositions." This deprivation began in childhood when, in contrast to the rough freedom granted little boys, young girls were taught to "dress up, sit still, and be pretty." Her natural ebullience "blasted, dwarfed, and perverted, in childhood; to just that extent must her womanhood, if ever attained, be imperfect."[22] The teacher and dress reformer Abba Gould Woolson argued that, in effect, invalidism was made intrinsic to women's social role in America. They had not only become prone to disease, but had learned to luxuriate in it. Women had to be reeducated to desire good health. "Disease must in time be considered as either a disgrace or a misfortune." As things stood then, girls ate rich and unnourishing food,

121

wore tight corsets, stayed up late at parties, crocheted, and dabbled at the piano instead of running and playing outside. "Thus we see that girls, from their childhood, have no proper means of unfolding and strengthening their physical natures."[23]

For the environmentalists the process of overcoming female sickliness was quite simple. "We should endeavor to remove the causes of evil," Dr. Smith argued, "by inducing mothers to rear their own children by means that nature has given them."[24] As Smith and the others presumed that women were by nature strong, correct education and the will to be healthy would serve to strip away false overlays of civilization in order to return girls to their good natural state.

Biological determinists, on the other hand, believed that women by nature were defined by physical characteristics and driven by powerful emotions verging on the pathological. Such advisors logically could place little hope in education. Unable or unwilling to face the implications of their own pessimism, even the biological determinists developed a concept of the will as the fool-proof governor of the ever-threatening emotions and bodily weaknesses. Thus in *The Coming Woman,* Lyman warned, "Woman must first control herself, before she can control others. She must learn to set the heel of Will on the head of Passion, and thus hold it in abeyance."[25] Women had to use their powers of will to stop their strong emotions from degenerating into debilitating nervous illness. "Better than any remedy is prevention, and, if the mind can exercise a curative influence over an unstrung nervous system, there is no doubt that, by means of proper physical, mental, and moral training, the predisposition to neuropathic complaints which specialists declare universal in women, may be very nearly extinguished."[26] S. Weir Mitchell's rest cure for nervously distraught women focused on breaking the spell of perfervid emotionalism: "For the nervous, strong emotions are bad or risky, and from violent mirth to anger all are to be sedulously set aside."[27] Mitchell put his faith in a kind of behavior modification in which the unhealthy emotions would be repressed by the "slow, steady, hopeful training of the will power through every-day effort."[28]

Clearly, this powerful will had to emanate from some source independent of the biological weaknesses that caused all the problems in the first place—and yet, the will was itself a product of evolution, a biological process. This inconsistency and overlapping of metaphysics and materialism strike the modern reader as illogical and unintentionally ironic, but for late Victorians belief in the power of the will was obviously a constructive way of coping with otherwise insuperable problems presented by biological materialism. Perhaps we can duplicate some of their unwillingness to submit to the consequences of determinism if we examine the attitudes of our culture toward the impact of heredity. We tend to hedge against the possibility of hereditarian determinism by insisting that some characteristics may be inherited but that others are totally induced by the environment, that whatever our inborn limitations may be, we should still strive to develop our talents to the fullest.

Will was the chief mechanism for freeing the self from the domination of determinist forces, but since individuals could not be expected to expend their limited fund of time and energy on every little choice that life presented, they had to render automatic their exercise of will. They needed to transform their conscious efforts at self-improvement into habit, freeing the will for new challenges. "The conscious energy of past function becomes the unconscious mechanism of present function, which thereupon is able to work without attention and almost without exertion," wrote Henry Maudsley in 1883. "Will loses its character, so to speak, in attaining to its unconscious perfection; and meanwhile the free, unattached, path-seeking consciousness, and will . . . the pioneers and perfecters of progress, are available to initiate new and to perfect old functions."[29] Habit was to be used to systematize moral behavior, to lead to that lifelong self-control and self-improvement the late Victorians considered so essential. "Whenever we do a wrong act, it becomes easier to do the same again, and our power of resisting temptation is lessened with each repetition of the act," admonished J. H. Kellogg, the sex and food purist of Battle Creek, Michigan, where the Seventh Day Adventist Sanitorium was located. "On the other hand, our resolution and ability to resist evil are strengthened each time we overcome a temptation."[30] Habit was far more fundamental to good health than any other factor, including medication, William A. Hammond stressed. "The proper regulation of the habits conduces more to mental and physical well-being than perhaps any other factor."[31] This stance placed the possibility of good health within the realm of individual self-control.

Habit altered mental structure, many scientists believed, through direct physical impact upon the brain. "Every state of ideational consciousness which is either very strong or is habitually repeated," William James wrote in *Popular Science Monthly* in 1887, "leaves an organic impression on the cerebrum."[32] Other writers described this imprinting upon the brain through habit as "probably a casting of some of the protoplasmic molecules into a particular form," and as "change . . . petrified in brain-structure."[33] Kellogg emphasized the negative argument that "every bad habit makes a scar upon the brain which sometimes requires many years to remove." Therefore, the malleability of youthful brain tissue argued for the urgency of instilling good habits in the young.[34] An extension of this perception of habit, in a pregenetic hereditarian era, was to view acquired habits as transmissible from parent to child. The demands for self-control were central to the individual as progenitor and not merely as independent moral agent. Temperance writers in particular were attracted to this guilt-inducing argument. Kellogg wrote, "We inherit our brains just as we do our faces, so, if a man spoils his brain with alcohol and gets an alcoholic appetite, his children will be likely to have unhealthy brains and an appetite for alcohol also, and may become drunkards."[35] Discussing the hereditarily acquired disposition to tubercular habits, Dr. J. M. W. Kitchen argued that one "habit that may be hereditary or acquired is slothfulness, which, if indulged in, must bring about a diseased condition in its possessor," leading as it did to "generally unhealthy and debilitated states of the body, in which state the lungs would offer a ready field of action for any special irritation."[36] The train of evil results from bad habits would be without end, reemerging in some dreadful form in unsuspecting descendants. Thus Dr. Ireneus Davis warned little girls, "Habits may even be transmitted to the third or fourth generation . . . even when they have not appeared in the intervening ones. So the habits that we are now forming will add to the happiness or misery of the world a hundred years from now."[37] Apparently, the future of the nation and the race depended upon the acquisition of good habits and the avoidance of bad ones.

William James insisted that habit was to be achieved only through action, that is, through motor effects rather than through mere resolution or feeling, and this was in keeping with one popular method designed to foster good habits, the physical culture movement. In 1890, the author of *A Natural Method of Physical Training* advised his readers that the healthy conduct of life required, among other actions, the conscious use of the right muscles. Later on, he assured them, the proper management of the correctly trained body would become largely involuntary and unconscious: "Our habits do more to form our bodies as well as our minds than the conscious efforts at improvement."[38] The physical culture movement, largely derived from Europe, had an earlier history in the United States, but was suddenly ubiquitous in late nineteenth-century America both in the form of competing systems of exercise and in the mania for sports. On one level, of course, the need for physical culture reflected an increasingly urban life-style and sedentary occupations which excluded regular physical exercise and included many temptations to bad habits and softness. The almost total lack of interest in encouraging sports and physical recreation among working-class people suggests that physical exercise was a way of reintroducing substitute physical labor into the lives of softening middle-class Americans.[39]

Like sex, physical culture was never celebrated for the

pure physical pleasure or joy to be derived from it, but because it served moral and social purposes. Systematic exercise seemed to offer an opportunity to regain control over the lazy body, but its adherents had even more grandiose pretensions for it: they saw it as the principal method to train body, mind, and will. It was no accident, then, that Dio Lewis, the transcendentalist food and sexual reformer, founded the first actual training school for the teaching of gymnastics in the public schools. Opened in the early 1860s, Lewis's Boston Normal Physical Training School produced in seven years 500 graduates to spread the gospel of physical exercise.[40] A fellow enthusiast, D. H. Jacques, in his book, *How to Grow Handsome,* originally published in 1859 and reprinted throughout the latter part of the nineteenth century, promised his readers perfection through mental and physical culture. Through correct exercise, he exhorted, "we may impart fresh vitality to the languid frame; give strength to the weak limb; substitute grace of motion for awkwardness; remodel the ill-formed body and homely features into symmetry and beauty, and postpone indefinitely the infirmities and deformities of age." And then he concluded, "If moral perfection be within the range of human capability, physical perfection, surely, must also be attainable."[41] By the end of the nineteenth century, transcendental optimism such as Jacques's was muted, and at least one observer, sated with the torrent of physical culturist "twaddle," sourly repudiated almost all exercise. Horatio C. Wood concluded with nasty wit that not only was exercise not "the grand panacea for all individual ills, as well as the hope of the perfection of the race," but that, in fact, those who exercise daily, such as farmers and laborers, "not only die as well as other people, but even appear to suffer nearly or quite as much during their earthly pilgrimage."[42] By the late nineteenth century, perfectionist claims may have been played down, but most physical culture writers still insisted that through the reintroduction of physical exertion to balance the mental, they had a key method by which to rescue a physically and morally flabby populace. Genevieve

126

Stebbens promised that her system of exercise would bring out "the potential of the body and the soul by bringing them into harmony," surely an alluring prospect both for the individual, and, after a debilitating period of political and industrial disharmony, for American society.[43]

Although their books are filled with suggestions for precise exercises, and for a variety of athletic equipment, all the physical culturists assumed that exercise had a higher purpose than the mere development of the body for its own sake. Strengthening the body would develop the mind, the character, and the will. As the mind, through the nervous system, permeated the entire body, the sound body in this reciprocal relationship was the responsive servant to the mind's commands. Carl Betz, superintendent of physical culture of the public schools of Kansas City, Missouri, set a double task for systematic exercise: developing children's bodies and improving discipline in the schools. In the frontispiece of his book, *A System of Physical Culture,* he stated that his purpose was "to unfold the natural and symmetrical beauty of the human body, making it fit and capable, in every phase of moral life, to adopt and carry out the will of its supreme master, the Mind."[44] John Boyle O'Reilly, one of the few advisors to be concerned with physical exercise for "the common man," defended the despised and feared working-class sport of boxing, pointing out that "there is character as well as strength in muscle; and little of either in flabbiness or lard."[45] Others agreed that the undisciplined and neglected body would abuse the soul and intellect. Charles W. Emerson, president of the Emerson College of Oratory in Boston, warned that the "constricted" body would lead to the "misrepresentation of the soul," that, "a Christian heart cannot express itself through a savage body." Thinking as well as feeling would be hindered by an inactive and inexpressive body, so that "although the body is the natural servant of the intellect, when contracted into the rebellious servant it will not respond to the intel-

127

lect."[46] Even those people who thought they were done with physical labor could not afford to ignore their bodies. To do the brain work that was characteristic of modern middle-class occupations and life-styles, the individual needed the cooperation of the body.

While bodily exercise was justified by its impact upon the mind, in turn the metaphor of exercise was extended to mental training by the physical culturists who sought to establish the prestige of physical exercise by linking it to mental discipline. This equation of the disciplines implied that life for most readers did not include natural exercise.[47] Dr. S. M. Barnett, who boasted that the New York City Board of Education had adopted his patented chest expander, insisted that "the physical, like the intellectual, requires systematic culture. Compare the action of study and we shall be convinced that it is a mental calisthenic developing by exercise the faculties and forces of the brain."[48] Mental, like physical training, had its rules—guides to behavior based upon natural law—which the physical culturists sought to tap. "There is a 'training' for the brain as well as for the body," Richard A. Proctor instructed the readers of *Popular Science Monthly,* "—a real physical training—depending, like bodily training, on rules as to nourishment, method of action, quantity of exercise, etc."[49] Mental and physical exercise were not merely parallel, but were parts of a whole. Overcoming obstacles in one meant increasing strength in both. A physical education instructor at Yale noted "the effect of exercise upon the character," arguing that "in all muscular exercise a certain amount of resistance had to be overcome, and the power which acts through the muscles to overcome this resistance is will-power. Development of strength is . . . development of will."[50]

According to these writers, physical culture had both concrete, physiological effects upon the brain and significant social implications for the nation. Exercise stimulated the circulation and purification of the blood, thus insuring the brain of an invigorated supply.[51] Strong muscles would mean strong nerves, an end to that encroaching American nervousness which, as we indicated in chapter 4, many writers feared as a major symptom of the decay wrought upon Americans by overcivilization.[52]

At the least, then, exercise was a means of warding off further disaster, further deterioration of already vulnerable nervous systems and flabby bodies. One physical culture writer insisted that gymnastics was necessary to compensate for "civilization . . . pursuit of artificial luxuries [and] creature comforts," while another thought that gymnastics and the accompanying inclination "to harden their bodies to the intemperance of the seasons, climates and elements, to hunger, thirst and fatigue" would make people impervious to most diseases.[53] But unlike the physicians, the neurophysiologists, the food reformers, and the sexual advisors, with their efforts to establish balances, to hold on moderately, writers about exercise never lost completely—or perhaps found anew—the perfectionist optimism that was more common to health writers of the earlier nineteenth century. They wrote expansively of the "development of physical powers," the possession of "maximum vigor," a "more perfect condition of physical health, exuberance of spirits, a clear brain and the energy inseparable from success in all enterprises."[54]

Such trumpetings might all be put down to entrepreneurial oversell by the purveyors of exercise systems and equipment, but what interests us is the more general emphasis on exercise for women, which from the 1830s was stressed as a means of helping women attain their natural potential. In 1829, Frances Wright's insistence that justice required the "fair and thorough development of all the faculties, physical, mental and moral" of women, was applied in her advocacy of the benefits of "wholesome exercise" being put within women's reach.[55] In concert with many other female cultural leaders, Elizabeth Cady Stanton at mid-century endorsed exercise for women, arguing that "physically as well as intellectually, it is *use* that produces growth and development."[56] By 1890, the engineer Edwin Checkley was telling women that by leading active lives, "their strength and endurance" would come "remarkably close to the strength and endurance of the other sex."[57] After having heard a woman physician lecture in the 1870s, the teen-aged Charlotte Perkins [Gilman] took to "every kind of attainable physical exercise . . . the beginning of a life-long interest in physical culture." She moved from the small to the large, from the physical to the moral, to a full "system of self-development," resulting in "many years of progressive improvement, physical and mental."[58]

For many writers the fully realized individual would be one who exercised his or her way to full vigor. Ed. James, the sporting journalist, drew this assumption to its logical conclusion by portraying the athlete as the physically perfect human being: "Winter's cold or summer's heat possess no fears for athletes, and statistics show that insanity seldom if ever happens to this class, who are better able to withstand reverses, adversity and sorrow."[59] In a presumably democratic, individualist society, such an emboldened individual was the chief social goal. The first annual catalogue of the Boston Normal School of Gymnastics stated as the school's aim: "a symmetrically developed form" directed toward creating individuals ready for "the various practical purposes life may demand," equipped with "self-reliance, self-control, courage, and a joyous disposition."[60] The individual thus prepared should be able to discover "strange countries," and with "a smack of Columbus about him" be eager to sail across alien oceans, Julian Hawthorne claimed in *Harper's Monthly* in 1884.[61] The late nineteenth century saw the rise of college football, "—a most manly game," in the words of one of its boosters. Here competition was raised to the pitch of "a battle in which courage and self-possession not only assured victory but safety," the football fan enthused.[62] Whether this was a moral equivalent to war, or a preparation for war, in what was, after all, a period of intense Western imperialism, is perhaps a moot point; but just as individuals were to gird themselves for battle, so the nation or race could be renewed through physical culture in preparation for worldwide conquests. "Physical exercise is destined to effect the regeneration of the Caucasian race," Bernarr A. McFadden trumpeted.[63]

The focus upon habit, as in our example of physical culture, was the optimistic side of the emphasis upon the will, although even the physical training boom produced anxiety that, as James C. Whorton puts it, the exercise which overcame "debility caused by slothfulness" would in turn produce "a new debility from over-exercise" on the part of people unable to control their tendencies to immoderation of exercise.[64] The darker underside was the haunting fear that the will would prove insufficient after all, and that the fearsome lower propensities would overwhelm the will, conquer, and rule the self. The theological notion of innate depravity no longer dominated late nineteenth-century American thought, and the psychological notion of unconscious drives had yet to gain ascendancy. Consequently, Americans' images of what lay beneath the human exterior were foggy; this very lack of clarity fed the advisors' fears of potential chaos.

Breakdown of the governing agency of the will could have anarchic implications for the unleashed self. If subversive elements such as alcohol, opium, lust, or hypnotism were to infiltrate the self, the will could be overthrown and the self ruined. "A gradual weakening of Volitional control," Carpenter admonished, would be the drunkard's downward path, "as the alcoholized blood takes more and more hold of the Brain." The debased drunkard would collapse as a human "when the government of the Will is completely overthrown, and the excited passions rage uncontrolled, the drunkard may be most truly said to be a madman . . . completely irresponsible for his actions . . . he has lost all power either of restraining his vehement impulses or of withdrawing himself from their influence."[65] Writing in gratitude to his physician, an ex-chloroform addict described his realization that his "pet habit" had been becoming his "tyrannical master" until the doctor helped him to recover his "self-respect" and "power of will."[66] An immoderate sexuality would also destroy the self. "There are some appetites that, when fully aroused, paralyze the will, and control of the whole being," one advisor instructed young girls. Sexual caresses could arouse the baser passions until "a moment arrives when the reason and will of both persons are suddenly overwhelmed by fierce lust and two lives are forever disgraced."[67]

In many aspects of involuntary behavior, the control of the will was threatened. For example, Hammond was wary of the welling up of dreams during sleep. "The emotions have full play, unrestrained by the Will, and governed only by the imagination. The Will or Volition is entirely suspended."[68] Perhaps the ordinary individual could do no more than be cognizant of the dangers of dreams, but he could avoid courting those states of heightened feeling or irrationalism represented by the then fashionable interest in hypnotism and spiritual trances in which the person was to give himself up to the dreamlike suspension of the will.[69] Degrading in itself, submission to mindlessness would finally warp the powers of judgment. Carpenter warned, "If the directing power of the Will be entirely suspended, the capability of correcting the most illusory ideas by an appeal to Common Sense is for the time annihilated."[70]

Loss of will carried to the extreme was defined as an essential characteristic of insanity. Those "lower mental functions" which were controlled by the will in a sane person, one physician wrote in *Popular Science Monthly*, would control the insane self, "expressed in delusions, hallucinations, wild and whirling words, and extravagant actions." This "impairment of will is . . . the universal element in insanity," as opposed to the legal distinction of knowing right from wrong.[71] Extreme emotionalism, by its nature unchecked by the will, was both a sign and a cause of insanity. "Undue excitement of the passions" or "violent anger" would produce "mental confusion," derangement of the functioning of certain organs, "a state of permanent irritability" which would render the brain "particularly liable to the inroads of functional disorders."[72]

Because the will was the highest human characteristic, the most recently evolved, it was also the most vulnerable to biological and cultural atavism. As Henry Maudsley said, "When the mind undergoes degeneration [will] is the first to show it, as it is the last to be restored when the disorder passes away."[73] Thus the entire ideological construct which culminated in the will was very fragile. Fear of disorder and chaos paralleled belief in self-control and the will. Perhaps evil resided in humankind's natural biological state and could not be uprooted. Will, a necessary dynamic element which could lead people to self-improvement, might amount only to whistling in the dark. Perpetual individual struggle, absolutely essential if the individual were to be truly lawful, might well prove insufficient.

Conclusion _____

Perhaps the naturally instructible, commonsensical will would allow the perplexed individual to skirt the limitations of the threatened body and mind. The bulk of the popular ideology we have analyzed seemed to plumb the larger questions of human-kind in nature and in civilization to no clear end, other, perhaps, than underlining a vision of ever-increasing troubles. Sickness and disorder, both personal and social, were widespread, and the ageless desire for balance and moderation was so weak a way to keep the threats at bay. Belief in the will was something of a leap in the dark toward higher, broader ground than that offered by advisors with their cautious offers of balance and stability. The opposite of such an assertion of will must have been depression, and depressives, of course, did not have the energy to write books cloaked with cheerful self-assertion (clothes meant to re-make the man or woman). Clearly, the will was desperately needed. Fundamentally, however, this advice literature which included positive thinking, did not add up to a boosterism of the self. Will was needed because anxiety was deep, because hygiene rules were limited as emotional remedies, and because the big questions about nature and civilization produced no satisfactory answers.

Within popular ideology of the self, one can discover ex-pressions of what James Gilbert, writing of work, calls the late nineteenth-century crisis of individualism in an antipathetic age.[1] In the new century, Gilbert argues, the Progressives made "gestures of resolution" focused less on the inner self as moral guardian than on the outer behaviorial self as conceived in so-cial settings. Whether batteries of psychological and intelli-gence tests, the construction of playgrounds, Taylorism, inves-tigative and regulatory agencies, and other Progressive devices amounted to coercive external social control or, as Paul Boyer has recently argued, to attempts to create a noncoercive envi-ronment to which the individual would willingly adjust himself, is an argument beyond the scope of this essay.[2] At any rate, the ground had shifted on which the individual and the community were engaged. The American individual conceptualized as a self, isolated before the bar of total and final judgment, of course, has continued until our day, but he or she, from the turn of the century, has at the same time been dealt with in a collective and often more dynamic framework.

Far from complete, the shift to a more collective, more process-oriented framework may have amounted only to those gestures of resolution as Gilbert writes, or to "awkward and hesitant compromises," as Daniel Rodgers concludes.[3] Indeed, much advice literature continued to employ language of static external law above social and personal constructs quite similar to those of the late nineteenth century. For example, the sociologist Luther Lee Bernard, writing in 1911, asserted, "Where a social fact is established it shall become as obligatory as the laws of astronomy or physics. The wilful disregard of the laws of health, of social hygiene, or public morality should have as little tolerance as a wilful disregard of the law of falling bodies when the question of this law has social consequences of equal importance."[4] Suprahistorical laws remained (and the destructive image of falling bodies is an interestingly vivid metaphor of destruction for lawbreaking), but now the stress was on social facts as opposed to laws of nature; social consequences as the basis of moral judgment.

As did law, which was reworked from nature to society, the will persisted as a central device, but now it could become, with the discovery of the unconscious, part of an abundant individual energy source, sometimes liberating, sometimes frightening, linked to a similarly ambiguous, dynamic society. The personal and social dangers of sexual repression, for example, rather than the fears of too much sex, were often expressed in at least avant garde advice literature and clinical psychology. In general, images of social abundance and the potential of finding collective means to overcome problems tilted the balance of possible gains and losses in the early twentieth century as compared with the *fin de siècle* we have analyzed. Yet metaphors of abundance, energy, sexual expression, and even play for relaxation rather than as moral gymnastics coexisted with a continuing demand for tightly governed individual self-improvement. Indeed, it would be useful to discover the degree to which personal and social engineering and problem-solving have spread, even in the new middle class, to the exclusion of the frightened inward-turning moral soldiery we have described.

The grasping, anxious American individual forever marches, perhaps stumbles would be better, out of soothing categories of abundance and social fit. Indeed, we are still living in an age where the self is threatened by social and final law, as in the late nineteenth century. General cultural malaise continues to be focused on explanations for the body and the mind, where, on balance, fragility rather than self-confidence characterizes the content of much ideological explanation. Writing in the *New Eng-*

land Journal of Medicine, Dr. Lewis Thomas, president of the Memorial Sloan-Kettering Cancer Center, concludes that not only are Americans "obsessed with health," but that this is the obsession of an ever-anxious individual feeling "fundamentally fragile, always on the verge of mortal disease, perpetually in need of support by health care professionals. . . . We do not seem to be seeking more exuberance in living as much as staving off failure, putting off dying. We are losing confidence in the human form." Dr. Thomas sees the concern with personal health, the fetish for jogging, tennis, health food, and vitamins as mechanisms which heighten narcissism, as means for leaving the social world behind. Thomas believes that medicine is improving, and that obsessive self-concern and belief in individual fragility is not merely incorrect, but socially harmful. "Indeed, we should be worrying that our preoccupation with personal health may be a symptom of copping out, an excuse for running upstairs to recline on a couch sniffing the air for contaminates, spraying the room with germicides, while just outside the whole of society is coming undone."[5]

A general sense that the world outside is coming undone is frequently related to the haunting fear that the body and the mind are fragile structures. The imperiled body is both metaphor and ideological focus. As E. D. Pellegrino writes, "Medicine is an exquisitely sensitive indicator of the dominant cultural characteristics of any era, for Man's behavior before the threats and realities of illness is necessarily rooted in the conception he has constructed of himself and his universe."[6] In many ways the decline of the 1970s from the half-stated programs of the 1960s was rather like the decline of the late nineteenth century from the more self-confident program of antebellum America. In the late nineteenth century, as now, the senses of potential chaos, in both the personal and social worlds, reverberated together in an ominous harmony. Nihilistic personal and social atonality were impermissible to late nineteenth-century Americans. All attempts at ordering devices were preferable to the possibility that there was no order at all. To have had meaning for a broad public, ideology on the body and the mind must have had to ring bells on many social and psychological levels: artificial, invented sets of ideas simply would not have achieved an appearance of order, except through some blatant and systematic coercion not present in late nineteenth-century America in the sector of ideology we are discussing.[7] There was a compelling need which led our ancestors to ask for blueprints to explain themselves to themselves. This demand, joined to responses to it, was one of the primary origins of authority in the late nineteenth-century American liberal capitalist world. The strident, often frightening appeal was to the harsh censor within the individual; it was not simply power imposed. Such liberal authority was far more powerful than that which any external legions might have provided.

What we have said concerning popular ideology found within the genre of advice literature about the body and the mind applies to other sectors of self and to other literary forms. Indeed, a great deal of excellent work has been done on nineteenth-century popular ideology concerning the soul, vocation, and personal surroundings, as found in sentimental fiction, domestic and architectural guides, and religious pamphlets, four other prevalent literary genres. We refer in particular to the work of Sacvan Bercovitch, Donald M. Scott, Kathryn Kish Sklar, Ann Douglas, and Gwendolyn Wright.[8] Each of these authors has sought to clarify the ideological content within a literary mode, to link the intellect and more originally the emotions, with the social setting. Moreover, each analyzes the development of a dominant middle-class world view which accompanied the construction of modern American capitalism. These studies, and we hope our own, serve as markers on the path toward a fuller analysis of the need for popular ideology and its construction and content, range and boundaries; as an analysis of one major means by which nineteenth-century American liberal-capitalist society was and was not integrated. It points to a reinvigoration of American intellectual history, which is now tending to become the study of the constructs in which disembodied and emotionally void intellectuals hold discourse with

139

each other.[9] It is a critique of all the discussions of "transcendence" in American Studies, as if in their creations artists somehow floated away from their persons and social contexts. In addition, insofar as certain social historians tend to discuss segregated fragments as if they were isolated, one from the other, and from power and authority in the society as a whole,[10] these studies are an effort to find some of the means by which a bourgeois hegemony tied those islands together in something increasingly approaching a national culture, with shared values, broadly middle class, such as those on the body and mind.

Perhaps the most urgent need now is to study ordinary people in nineteenth-century America, not merely in materially defined and circumscribed fragments, as workers and unionists, as shop clerks and craftsmen, as blacks or ethnics, as voters or neighborhood residents, but also as fearful, resentful, hopeful aspirants to widely diffused symbols of legitimacy, first those of a noble, redeemed, moderately prosperous yeomanry, and later those of a materially acquisitive, security-grasping urban "middling" class. The "reality" of the "myth" was in consciousness, and must be tested there whatever its material "reality." Conjointly one might discuss anew the ways in which American leaders have felt compelled to appear part of this middling way. The attempt to enter and dominate this vast middle ground could well be analyzed in periods of crisis as well as in periods of relative calm, in political pamphlets as well as in advice literature and the other manners we have just mentioned.[11]

Indeed, the study of popular ideology should help erase the artificial line between that which is political and that which is apolitical, between formal politics and the politics of everyday life. In a similar manner, it should blur the supposed distinctions in historical analysis between thought and emotion (the rational and the irrational), formal logic and the logic of experience.

Yet the study of the growth of middle-class hegemony should not be a means of falling back into cultural homogenization or American history as blessed consensus. Disparities in power relationships were reinforced in this process of ideological development. Also, popular ideology always included dispute, a sense of insufficiency and of the void. This was no bland, frictionless blending and arbitration, but a rough, often fearsome jostling. Also, we have tried to be quite specific about genres, subject matter, and eras in which general sets of beliefs about the body and the mind were reformed. This was a period of decline from a more stridently hopeful period of beliefs about the self, concurrent to a time of greatly unsettling social change, of invasions on the more intimate as well as on the social level. The sense of real work and production, of ever-growing or even stable, family and community was being lost, and the structures of late capitalism appeared everywhere in alien, invading forms. The shifting twentieth-century order was to be replete with contradictions and insufficiency amidst its considerable production of abundance and order. Poised at the end of the nineteenth century, middling Americans were filled with morbid symptomology balanced by hope for birth of the new. Yet those symptoms indicated a profound and ineradicable personal and social malaise, and a social and economic order that was to be propped up more than renewed. The tenacity of emphasis on the will to overcome the forever fragile self was as profound as the basic economic and social forms have proven to be. Hence popular ideology covering the self is not a secondary and dispensable set of fads, but a deep and necessary series of ordering devices. Whether the need for ideology or the shapes of this one are cause for regret is another question, but this sector of ideology is no more nor less artificial than the culture from which it grows, and to which it bears witness.

ABBREVIATIONS————

PSM Popular Science Monthly

JNMD Journal of Nervous and Mental Disease

AJO American Journal of Obstetrics and Diseases of Women and
Children

JSH Journal of Social History

JHM Journal of the History of Medicine and Allied Sciences

BHM Bulletin of the History of Medicine

142

Notes _____

Making Sense of Self

1. Quoted in Roberta J. Park, " 'Embodied Selves': The Rise and Development of Concern for Physical Education, Active Games and Recreation for American Women, 1776–1865," *Journal of Sport History* 5 (Summer 1978): 37n.

2. George M. Beard, *Our Home Physician* (New York, 1870), pp. iii–xxi.

3. Mary Douglas, *Natural Symbols* (New York, 1970), pp. 98–99; Charles Rosenberg, "Science, Society and Social Thought," reprinted in *No Other Gods, On Science and American Social Thought* (Baltimore, 1976), p. 10.

4. John B. Blake, "Health Reform," in Edwin S. Gaustad, ed., *The Ride of Adventism, Religion and Society in Mid-Nineteenth-Century America* (New York, 1974), pp. 30–31.

5. James C. Whorton, "The Hygiene of the Wheel: An Episode in Victorian Sanitary Science," *BHM* 52 (Spring 1978): 61.

6. For a recent analysis of the antebellum health-reform movement, replete with historiographical information, see Regina Markell Morantz, "Making Women Modern: Middle Class Women and Health Reform in Nineteenth-Century America," *JSH* 10 (Summer 1977): 490–507. Other useful introductions include John Blake, "Health Reform"; Stephen W. Nissenbaum, "Careful Love: Sylvester Graham and the Emergence of Victorian Sexual Theory in America, 1830–1840" (Ph.D. diss., University of Wisconsin, 1968); Richard Shryock, "Sylvester Graham and the Popular Health Movement," *Medicine in America: Historical Essays* (Baltimore, 1966), pp. 111–25; James C. Whorton, "Christian Physiology: William Alcott's Prescription for the Millennium," *BHM* 49 (Winter 1975): 466–81; Lewis Perry, " 'Progress, not Pleasure, is Our Aim': The Sexual Advice of an Ante-Bellum Radical [Henry Wright]," *JSH* 12 (Spring 1979): 354–66; and Ronald G. Walters, *American Reformers: 1815–1869* (New York, 1978). Michael Fellman has discussed some ambiguities latent in the antebellum sense of moral totality in *The Unbounded Frame: Freedom and Community in Nineteenth-Century American Utopianism* (Westport, Conn., 1973).

7. S. P. Fullinwider, "Insanity as the Loss of Self: The Moral Insanity Controversy Revisited," *BHM* 49 (Spring 1975): 93.

8. Augustus K. Gardner, *Conjugal Sins: Against the Laws of Life and Health* (New York, 1870), p. 180; A. H. Guernsey and Ireneus P. Davis, *Health at Home* (New York, 1884), p. 116.

9. Blake, "Health Reform," p. 47.

10. Guenter B. Risse, "Introduction," in Guenter B. Risse et al., eds., *Medicine Without Doctors: Home Health Care in American History* (New York, 1977), p. 1.

11. Ronald L. Numbers, "Do-It-Yourself the Sectarian Way," in *Medicine Without Doctors,* pp. 51–54.

12. John Blake, "From Buchan to Fishbein: The Literature of Domestic Medicine," in *Medicine Without Doctors,* p. 28.

13. Blake, "Health Reform," pp. 41–43.

14. Regina Markell Morantz, "Nineteenth-Century Health Reform and Women: A Program of Self-Help," in *Medicine Without Doctors,* p. 78.

15. Joseph Kett, *Formation of the American Medical Profession* (New Haven, 1968).

16. William Workman, "The Progress of Medical Science," *Medical Communications of the Massachusetts Medical Society* 8 (1854): 291–96, quoted in Blake, "Health Reform," pp. 43–44.

17. Blake, "From Buchan to Fishbein," p. 29.

18. George Rosen, *A History of Public Health* (New York, 1958), p. 341; William G. Rothstein, *American Physicians in the Nineteenth Century* (Baltimore, 1972), pp. 252–58.

19. Daniel T. Rodgers, *The Work Ethic in Industrial America* (Chicago, 1978), p. 21. Walt Whitman Rostow describes the transformation very well, calling it the "maturation of the economy," rather than "late capitalism," in *The Stages of Economic Growth: A Non-Communist Manifesto* (London, 1960), pp. 70–73.

20. For an analysis of the outside agitator as a prototype in British and American strike literature, see Anita Clair Fellman, "The Fearsome Necessity: Nineteenth-Century British and American Strike Novels" (Ph.D. diss., Northwestern University, 1969).

21. For a compelling interpretation of this period, see Robert H. Wiebe, *The Search for Order, 1877–1920* (New York, 1967), pp. 11–110.

22. Stephen Freedman, "The Baseball Fad in Chicago, 1865–1870: An Exploration of the Role of Sport in the Nineteenth-Century City," *Journal of Sport History* 5 (Summer 1978): 43.

23. Andrew Nebinger, *Criminal Abortion: Its Extent and Prevention* (Philadelphia, 1870), p. 16.

24. James B. Gilbert, *Work Without Salvation, America's Intellectuals and Industrial Alienation 1880–1910* (Baltimore, 1977); Rodgers, *Work Ethic.*

25. Rodgers, *Work Ethic,* pp. 10–11. Rodgers reports that whereas the country's population a little more than tripled between 1860 and 1920, the volume of manufactured goods produced increased between twelvefold and fourteenfold. *Work Ethic,* p. 27.

26. *The Works of William E. Channing, D.D.,* 12th complete ed., 6 vols. (Boston, 1853), 5:158, quoted in Rodgers, *Work Ethic,* p. 10.

27. Census Office, United States Department of the Interior, *Report on the Population of the United States at the Eleventh Census, 1890* (Washington, D.C., 1895), p. 11.

28. S. Weir Mitchell, *Wear and Tear or Hints for the Overworked* (Philadelphia, 1871), pp. 5–6. Also see Harry Kane, *Drugs That Enslave: The Opium, Morphine, Chloral, and Hasheesh Habits* (Philadelphia, 1881), p. 17; R. V. Pierce, *The People's Common-Sense Medical Adviser* (Buffalo, 1889), p. 283; Freedman, "The Baseball Fad in Chicago," p. 47; Daniel Horowitz, "Consumption and Its Discontents: Simon N. Patten, Thorstein Veblen, and George Gunton," *Journal of American History* 67 (September 1980): 301–17. The difficulty of assessing productivity in service occupations continues to this day, and is still a source of anxiety for some white-collar workers. Writing in 1978, Robert Schrank, union official

and former machinist, remembers that in addition to the sense of freedom he felt at his release from the externally imposed discipline of the
plant, there was also a certain guilt: "I found I had a sort of subconscious
continuing concern that I was no longer productive, for what I was doing
was no longer measurable. How was I to know whether I was productive?
. . . Since I left the shop floor, I have never been able to answer that
question satisfactorily for myself. . . ." Robert Schrank, *Ten Thousand
Working Days* (Cambridge, Mass., 1978), p. 93; also see pp. 170–72.
Similar anxieties run through Sara Ruddick and Pamela Daniels, eds.,
*Working It Out: 23 Women Writers, Artists, Scientists, and Scholars Talk About
Their Lives and Work* (New York, 1977).

29. Mitchell, *Wear and Tear,* p. 10; J. S. Jewell, "Introductory,"
JNMD 1 (January 1874): 70–73; George M. Beard, *Eating and Drinking*
(New York, 1871), p. 127; P. J. Higgins, "Study-Physiologically Consid-
ered," *PSM* 24 (March 1884): 640; Rodgers, *Work Ethic,* pp. 105–6.

30. Julia and Annie Thomas, *Psycho-Physical Culture* (New York,
1892), p. 2; also see Richard A. Proctor, *Strength, How to Get Strong, and
Keep Strong* (London, 1889), pp. 2–5. Proctor was an assuager of the
uneasy, an apologist for the successful.

31. Mary Putnam Jacobi, "Modern Female Invalidism," in *A
Pathfinder in Medicine* (New York, 1925), p. 482; Augustus Hoppin, *A
Fashionable Sufferer* (Boston, 1883), pp. 14–16.

32. James C. Reed, *Private Vice to Public Virtue, Birth Control in
America, 1830 to the Present* (New York, 1978), p. 17.

33. Ibid., pp. x–xi.

34. In *The History of Sexuality: Volume I, An Introduction* (New York,
1978), pp. 81–91, Michel Foucault psychoanalyzes modern scholars
who, according to Foucault, need for their own purposes to project a
simplified, unified version of authority onto an especially conscious
group of paternal leaders, at the expense of a more subtle questioning
of order-giving and receiving.

35. Quentin Hoare and Geoffrey Nowell Smith, eds. and trans.,
Selections from the Prison Notebooks of Antonio Gramsci (New York, 1971), pp.
57–58. Three good introductions to Gramsci's ideas are Gwyn A. Williams, "The Concept of 'Egemonia' in the Thought of Antonio Gramsci:
Some Notes on Interpretation," *Journal of the History of Ideas* 22 (October
1960): 586–99; Thomas R. Bates, "Gramsci and the Theory of
Hegemony," *Journal of the History of Ideas* 36 (April 1975): 351–66; and
Perry Anderson, "The Antimonies of Antonio Gramsci," *New Left Review*
100 (November 1976): 5–78. Two helpful biographies are John M. Cammett, *Antonio Gramsci and the Origins of Italian Communism* (Palo Alto, Calif.,
1967); and the more personal Guiseppe Fiori, *Antonio Gramsci: Life of a*

Revolutionary (1965; London, 1970). In an American context, see Eugene D. Genovese's essay on Cammett, "On Antonio Gramsci," reprinted in *In Red and Black* (New York, 1971), pp. 391–422; and Aileen S. Kraditor's seminal essay, "American Historians on Their Radical Heritage," *Past and Present* 56 (August 1972): 136–53.

36. Erik H. Erikson, *Young Man Luther: A Study in Psychoanalysis and History* (New York, 1962), p. 14. Erikson's work is, of course, well known, and the book on Luther, as well as *Childhood and Society*, 2d ed. (New York, 1963), are the best starting places. Two less known essays by Erikson are especially valuable in defining his use of ideology: "Wholeness and Totality," in Carl J. Friedrich, ed., *Totalitarianism* (Cambridge, Mass., 1953), pp. 156–71, and *The Problem of Ego Identity: Identity and the Life Cycle, Psychological Issues* 1 (New York, 1959): 101–64.

37. This argument about ideology, employing Gramsci and Erikson, is fleshed out in Michael Fellman, "Approaching Popular Ideology in Nineteenth-Century America," *Historical Reflections* 6 (Winter 1979): 321–33.

38. Charles E. Rosenberg has argued recently that nineteenth-century American hospitals can be analyzed as battlegrounds for conflicting social values, in "And Heal the Sick: The Hospital and the Patient in Nineteenth-Century America," *JSH* 10 (June 1977): 428. This essay is one of a very useful set of articles devoted to the social history of medicine in the June 1977 issue of the *Journal of Social History*.

39. Herbert Spencer was the grand scientific-cultural synthesizer to many late Victorians, and the self-educated freethinker E. L. Youmans started *Popular Science Monthly* in part to bring Spencer to Americans. But the magazine broadened into a general attempt to join modern science to other middle-class modes of analysis, and Youmans enlisted a wide variety of scientific writers in a popularizing sense of task they all shared. See Robert C. Bannister, *Social Darwinism: Science and Myth in Anglo-American Thought* (Philadelphia, 1979), pp. 68–76; John Fiske, *Edward Livingston Youmans* (New York, 1894).

40. During this period, for example, the rigorously trained Viennese neurologist Sigmund Freud tried hydrotherapy, electrical farradization, massage, and the S. Weir Mitchell rest cure (which we discuss in chapter 7) before going on to develop psychoanalysis. Cf. Richard Wollheim, *Freud* (London, 1971), p. 24.

41. Hugh L. Hodge, *Foeticide, or Criminal Abortion: A Lecture Introductory to the Course on Obstetrics, and Diseases of Women and Children* (Philadelphia, 1869), pp. 9, 35–36.

42. Ann Douglas, *The Feminization of American Culture* (New York, 1977).

43. Barbara G. Rosenkrantz, "Cart Before the Horse: Theory, Practice and Professional Image in American Public Health, 1870–1920," *JHM* 29 (January 1974): 55; also see Gerald E. Markowitz and David Rosner, "Doctors in Crisis: Medical Education and Medical Reform During the Progressive Era, 1895–1915," in Susan Reverby and David Rosner, eds., *Health Care in America: Essays in Social History* (Philadelphia, 1979), pp. 185–205, for an indication that physicians' state of disorganization and marginal social position persisted somewhat beyond the period with which we are dealing.

The Healthy Self

1. Russell T. Trall, *The Hygienic System* (Battle Creek, Mich., 1872), pp. 5, 10–11; also see W. W. Hall, *Health at Home or Hall's Family Doctor* (Springfield, Mass., 1882), p. 304.

2. J. R. Black, *The Ten Laws of Health or How Disease Is Produced and Can Be Prevented* (Philadelphia, 1885), p. 29; Felix I. Oswald, "Physical Education," *PSM* 18 (January 1881): 303–4.

3. W. W. Hall, *The Guide-Board to Health, Peace, and Competence* (Springfield, Mass., 1869), p. 403.

4. Ronald L. Numbers, *Prophetess of Health: A Study of Ellen G. White* (New York, 1976), pp. 46, 61.

5. Martin Luther Holbrook, *Hygiene of the Brain and Nerves and the Cure of Nervousness* (New York, 1878), p. 61; Charles Rosenberg, "Science, Society and Social Thought," reprinted in *No Other Gods, On Science and American Social Thought* (Baltimore, 1976), p. 11; also see Ireneus P. Davis, *Hygiene for Girls* (New York, 1883), p. 118.

6. Felix L. Oswald, *Physical Education* (New York, 1882), p. 103.

7. Black, *The Ten Laws of Health*, p. 22.

8. Thomas H. Huxley and W. J. Youmans, *The Elements of Physiology and Hygiene: A Textbook for Educational Institutions* (New York, 1876), p. 347. For a useful depiction of the two magnets of primitivism and progress through science, see James C. Whorton, " 'Tempest in a Flesh-Pot': The Formulation of a Physiological Rationale for Vegetarianism," in Judith Walzer Leavitt and Ronald L. Numbers, eds., *Sickness and Health in America: Readings in the History of Medicine and Public Health* (Madison, Wis., 1978), pp. 315–30.

9. Edward Spencer, "The Philosophy of Good Health," *Scribner's Monthly* 4 (October 1871): 592; William James, *Talks to Teachers on Psychology: And to Students on Some of Life's Ideals* (1899) (reprint ed., New York, 1958), p. 45.

10. Felix L. Oswald, "Instinct as a Guide to Good Health," *PSM* 28 (February 1886): 518.

11. H. H. Kane, "A Hashish House in New York," *Harper's Monthly* 67 (November 1883): 944–49, reprinted in H. Wayne Morgan's fascinating collection *Yesterday's Addicts, American Society and Drug Abuse, 1865–1920* (Norman, Okla., 1974), pp. 159–70.

12. Dio Lewis, *Our Digestion; or My Jolly Friend's Secret* (Philadelphia, 1872), pp. 246, 256. Lewis's Spartan diet had the additional advantage of rationalizing the financial limits of the poor, much as does that of current dieticians who have suddenly discovered the problem of protein oversupply, just as meat prices have gone beyond the means of millions of Americans on limited incomes.

13. Oswald, *Physical Education*, p. 58.

14. Whorton, " 'Tempest in a Flesh-Pot,' " pp. 321, 325.

15. George M. Beard, *Eating and Drinking* (New York, 1871), pp. 58–59, 85–86, 91–96; and the same author's *Our Home Physician* (New York, 1870), pp. 167–70; Eliza B. Lyman, *The Coming Woman or the Royal Road to Perfection, A Series of Lectures* (Lansing, Mich., 1880), p. 120.

16. J. Leonard Corning, *Brain Rest* (New York, 1885), p. 29.

17. Abba Gould Woolson, *Women in American Society* (Boston, 1873), pp. 193–211.

18. Holbrook, *Hygiene of the Brain*, pp. 101, 151–272. This statement presumes that honest competition was the norm and leaves open the question of how a fellow businessman could handle the Jay Goulds of that world.

19. Edward Bayard, "Homeopathy as a Science," *PSM* 23 (October 1883): 738–41.

20. Ed. James, *How to Acquire Health, Strength and Muscle* (New York, 1877), p. 9; also see Joseph L. Hutchinson, *A Treatise on Physiology and Hygiene* (New York, 1892), p. 36.

21. W. W. Hall, *Health by Good Living* (New York, 1875), p. 53. For other vivid characterizations of "Cadaverous" vegetarians and Falstaffian flesh eaters, see Whorton, "Tempest," in Leavitt and Numbers, *Sickness and Health*, p. 318.

22. Dio Lewis, *Talks About People's Stomachs* (Boston, 1870), p. 95.

23. Corning, *Brain Rest*, p. 20; S. Weir Mitchell, *Wear and Tear or Hints for the Overworked* (Philadelphia, 1871), pass.; W. W. Hall, *Health and Disease as Affected by Constipation and Its Unmedicinal Cure* (New York, 1870), p. 71; Hall, *Guide-Board*, p. 140; Davis, *Hygiene for Girls*, p. 110. We would speculate that one of Davis's concerns stemmed from his associating anal and sexual functions, more particularly that he feared full bowels

would bring blood into the loins, thereby increasing sexual sensitivity and the inclination to masturbate.

24. A. H. Guernsey and Ireneus P. Davis, *Health at Home* (New York, 1884), p. 116; W. W. Hall, *Fun Better Than Physic; or Everybody's Life-Preserver* (Springfield, Mass., 1871), p. 49. Also see Holbrook, *Hygiene of the Brain*, p. 63.

25. "Hypochondria," *Godey's Lady Book and Magazine* 99 (August 1879): 184 (hereafter cited as *Godey's*); Hall, *Guide-Board*, p. 112.

26. L. M. Marston, *Essentials of Modern Healing* (Boston, 1887), p. 90; also see Gail Thain Parker, *Mind Cure in New England: From the Civil War to World War One* (Hanover, N.H., 1973); Stephen Gottschalk, *The Emergence of Christian Science in American Religious Life* (Berkeley, Calif., 1973); Raymond J. Cunningham, "From Holiness to Healing: The Faith Cure in America, 1872–1892," *Church History* 43 (December 1974): 499–513; Donald B. Meyer, *The Positive Thinkers: A Study of the American Quest for Health, Wealth and Personal Power from Mary Baker Eddy to Norman Vincent Peale* (Garden City, N.Y., 1965).

27. Dr. Humboldt advertised in *Harper's Weekly, Godey's,* and the New York *Tribune* that his cure-all would banish: "General debility, Mental and Physical Depression, Imbecility, Determination of the Blood to the Head, Confused Ideas, Hysteria, General Irritability, Restlessness and Sleeplessness at Night, Absence of Muscular Efficiency, Loss of Appetite, Dyspepsia, Emaciation, Low Spirits, Disorganization or Paralysis of the Organs of Generation, Palpitation of the Heart." Quoted in James Harvey Young, *The Toadstool Millionaires, A Social History of Patent Medicines in America Before Federal Regulation* (Princeton, N. J., 1961), p. 117.

28. Richard H. Shryock, "Sylvester Graham and the Popular Health Movement, 1830–1870," in *Medicine in Modern America, Historical Essays* (Baltimore, 1966), p. 120; Stephen Nissenbaum, "Careful Love; Sylvester Graham and the Emergence of Victorian Sexual Theory in America, 1830–1840" (Ph.D. diss., University of Wisconsin, 1968).

29. Frederik A. P. Barnard, "The Germ Theory of Disease and Its Relation to Hygiene" (1873), reprinted in Gert H. Brieger, ed., *Medical America in the Nineteenth Century, Readings from the Literature* (Baltimore, 1972), p. 292; Huxley and Youmans, *Elements of Physiology and Hygiene*, p. 349. According to John Harley Warner, many orthodox physicians accepted elements of the natural cure argument, but could not make it the exclusive base of their practice, as total nonintervention would render physicians superfluous. The physician observed nature, but intervened when necessary. "The Nature Trusting Heresy: American Physicians and the Concept of the Healing Power of Nature in the

1850s and 1860s," *Perspectives in American History* 11 (1977–78), pp. 291–324.

30. William H. Welch, "Considerations Concerning Some External Sources of Infection in Their Bearing on Preventive Medicine," *Science* 14 (1889): 71.

31. W. G. Thompson, "The Present Aspect of Medical Education," *PSM* 27 (September 1886): 590.

32. Black, *The Ten Laws of Health,* frontispiece.

The Unhealthy Self

1. W. W. Hall, *Fun Better Than Physic, or Everybody's Life-Preserver* (Springfield, Mass., 1871), p. 7; also see Eli F. Brown, *Sex and Life: The Physiology and Hygiene of the Sexual Organization* (Chicago, 1891), p. 7.

2. John D. Steele, *Hygienic Physiology* (New York, 1884), p. 232.

3. Frederik A. P. Barnard, "The Germ Theory of Disease and Its Relation to Hygiene" (1873), reprinted in Gert H. Breiger, ed., *Medical America in the Nineteenth Century, Readings from the Literature* (Baltimore, 1972), pp. 279–80; also see J. R. Black, *The Ten Laws of Health or How Disease is Produced and Can Be Prevented* (Philadelphia, 1872), p. 15; John Dye, *Painless Childbirth; or Healthy Mothers and Healthy Children,* 2d ed. (Silver Creek, N.Y. 1882), p. 7.

4. Black, *The Ten Laws of Health,* p. 24.

5. Leonard Corning, *Brain Exhaustion* (New York, 1884), pp. 182–83. Where one writer wanted to cut down to two meals and drinking water, another warned about the sour, depressing results of an underfed stomach. There was not always consensus as to what constituted immoderation. Dio Lewis, *Our Digestion, or My Jolly Friend's Secret* (Philadelphia, 1872), pass.; W. W. Hall, *Health by Good Living* (New York, 1875), p. 27; also see Thomas J. Huxley and W. J. Youmans, *The Elements of Physiology and Hygiene: A Textbook for Educational Institutions* (New York, 1876), p. 436; "How People Become Ill," *Godey's* 97 (March 1878): 261.

6. J. H. Kellogg, *Second Book on Physiology and Hygiene* (Philadelphia, 1894), pp. 227–28; Horatio C. Wood, *Brain-Work and Over-Work* (Philadelphia, 1880), pp. 54–58; George L. Austin, *Perils of American Womanhood, or a Doctor's Talk with Maiden, Wife, and Mother* (Boston, 1883), pp. 54–55. L. J. Rather gives examples of earlier beliefs of this interconnection in *Mind and Body in Eighteenth Century Medicine* (Berkeley, Calif., 1965), p. 8.

7. For an excellent discussion of the development and application of American vitalist theories, see Joseph F. Kett, *The Formation of the American Medical Profession, The Role of Institutions, 1780–1860* (New

Haven, 1968), pp. 133–39; also see Stanley W. Jackson, "Force and Kindred Notions in Eighteenth Century Neurophysiology, and Medical Psychology," *BHM* 44 (September, November 1970): 397–410; 539–54.

8. Edward Bayard, "Homeopathy as a Science," *PSM* 23 (October 1883): 732–33; also see James Harvey Young, *The Toadstool Millionaires, A Social History of Patent Medicine in America Before Federal Regulation* (Princeton, N.J., 1961), p. 151, and Martin Kaufman, *Homeopathy in America: The Rise and Fall of a Medical Heresy* (Baltimore, 1971). The effectiveness of immunization was to the homeopaths clear proof of their theory. For the continuing impact of homeopathic assumptions on folk medicine, see Wayland Hand, "Folk Medical Magic and Symbolism in the West," in Austin and Alta Fife and Harvey M. Glassie, eds., *Forms upon the Frontier: Folklife and Folk Arts in the United States,* Monographic Series (Logan, Utah, 1969), 16:103–18.

9. R. T. Trall, *Digestion and Dyspepsia* (New York, 1873), p. 12; also see Harvey B. Weiss and Howard R. Kemble, *The Great American Water Cure Craze: A History of Hydropathy in the United States* (Trenton, N. J., 1967).

10. Edward B. Foote, Jr., *Plain Home Talk* (New York, 1883), p. 26; also see George M. Beard and A. D. Rockwell, *On the Medical and Surgical Uses of Electricity* (New York, 1891); William A. Hammond, *Sexual Impotence in the Male and Female* (Detroit, 1887), p. 304. Interestingly enough, some spiritualists shared the notion of vital electrical force although their therapy was spiritual. Cf. Charles O. Sahler, *Psychic Life and Laws, or the Operations and Phenomena of the Spiritual Element in Man* (New York, 1901), pp. 137–38.

11. Nathan Allen, "The Law of Human Increase," *PSM* 22 (November 1882): 42.

12. J. H. Kellogg, *Plain Facts for Old and Young* (Burlington, Iowa, 1889), p. 119; S. Pancoast, *Boyhood's Perils and Manhood's Curse: A Handbook for the Father, Mother, Son and Daughter* (Philadelphia, 1873), pp. 31–32.

13. D. H. Jacques, *How to Grow Handsome* (New York, 1890), p. 58.

14. Samuel W. Gross and A. Haller Gross, eds., *Autobiography of Samuel D. Gross, M.D.,* 2 vols. (Philadelphia, 1887), 1: 7–8; also see George Wilson, *How to Live, or Health and Healthy Homes* (Philadelphia, 1882), p. 67.

15. John B. Blake, "From Buchan to Fishbein: The Literature of Domestic Medicine," in Guenter B. Risse et al., eds., *Medicine Without Doctors* (New York, 1977), p. 16.

16. George Rosen, *A History of Public Health* (New York, 1958),

p. 288; also see Wilson, *How to Live,* p. 68. Public health theories led to collective, often political, action. Miasmatists built sewer systems, purified water supplies, and drained swamps, while contagionists provided for widespread quarantines. A thorough case study is John Duffy's *A History of Public Health in New York City,* 2 vols. (New York, 1968, 1974).

17. Abraham Rothstein, *American Physicians in the Nineteenth Century* (Baltimore, 1972), pp. 252–72. The first truly useful new application of bacteriological theory came in surgery. Lister's initial bulky, wet, antiseptic techniques caused much scorn among American physicians and surgeons who became converted only by the aseptic techniques dating from the 1880s. Inoculation for many diseases previously responsible for high mortality became the second major bacteriological therapeutic application.

18. Henry Thompson, "The Present Aspect of Medical Education," *PSM* 27 (September 1885): 590. For the lurid reaction of the Kansas country doctor upon first seeing bacteria isolated under a microscope, see Thomas N. Bonner, *The Kansas Doctor: A Century of Pioneering* (Lawrence, Kans., 1959), p. 58. In our own time, widespread acceptance of the theory of carcinogens seems to be playing a similar role in medical and popular attitudes. This idea has also refined theory without presenting therapeutics.

19. Young, *The Toadstool Millionaires,* pp. 144–62.

20. Richard H. Shryock, "The Interplay of Social and Internal Factors in Modern Medicine," in *Medicine in America* (Baltimore, 1966), pp. 324–25.

21. Henry Gradle, *Bacteria and the Germ Theory of Disease* (Chicago, 1883), pp. 210, 212.

22. Charles M. Barrows, *Facts and Fictions of Mental Healing* (Boston, 1887), p. 163.

23. Charles Rosenberg, "The Bitter Fruit: Heredity, Disease, and Social Thought," reprinted in *No Other Gods: On Science and American Social Thought* (Baltimore, 1976), pp. 25–34.

24. George M. Beard, *Our Home Physician* (New York, 1870), pp. 383–84. Beard is, however, one of the very few to indicate that "good qualities are just as liable to inheritance as bad ones" (p. 385).

25. J. M. French, "Infant Mortality and the Environment," *PSM* 34 (December 1888): 222–23.

26. J. R. Black, "Removal of Inherited Tendencies to Disease," *PSM* 15 (August 1879): 433, 435; also see Henry Maudsley's books, *Responsibility in Mental Disease* (New York, 1874), p. 283, and *Body and Mind* (New York, 1875), pp. 68–69. Prohibitionists were often drawn to this logic, for not only would the fatal drop plunge naturally weak in-

dividuals constitutionally incapable of temperate imbibing into personal degradation, but it would surely undermine all heritable prospects for future generations. See R. T. Trall, *The Mother's Hygienic Handbook* (New York, 1874), p. 12; T. D. Crothers, "New Facts in Alcoholic Heredity," *PSM* 34 (February 1889): 524.

27. Clement Hammond, "The Prolongation of Human Life," *PSM* 34 (November 1888): 100.

Brain and Mind in Sickness and in Health

1. J. Milner Fothergill, "The Mental Aspects of Ordinary Disease," *PSM* 6 (March 1875): 562; for a modern analysis of this stance toward insanity, see Norman Dain, *Concepts of Insanity in the United States, 1789–1865* (New Brunswick, N.J., 1964), p. 66.

2. Editor's Table, "The Practical Study of Mind," *PSM* 20 (February 1882): 555; also see Alexander Bain, *Mind and Body* (New York, 1873), pp. 41, 130.

3. Henry S. Drayton and James McNeill, *Brain and Mind* (New York, 1880), pp. 284–85. For another late nineteenth-century restatement of phrenology, see Nelson Sizer, *40 Years of Phrenology* (New York, 1891). The best modern monograph on American phrenology remains John D. Davies, *Phrenology: Fad and Science* (New Haven, 1955).

4. E. L. Youmans, "Editor's Table: The Relation of Body and Mind," *PSM* 4 (November 1873): 111; also see M. Allen Starr, "The Old and the New Phrenology," *PSM* 35 (October 1889): 730. The development of British scientific study of the brain is carefully dissected in Robert M. Young, *Mind, Brain and Adaptation in the Nineteenth Century: Cerebral Localization from Gall to Ferrier* (Oxford, 1970).

5. H. Hughes Bennett, "Hygiene in the Higher Education of Women," *PSM* 16 (February 1880): 523.

6. Joseph Simms, "Human Brain Weights," *PSM* 31 (July 1887), 355–59. Interestingly, the patriotic Simms found that American blacks, while having smaller brains than whites, had larger brains than black Africans, due to the fact that colder climates led to heavier brains. Antebellum American uses of such scientific supports for racism are analyzed in William Stanton, *The Leopard's Spots: Scientific Attitudes Toward Race in America, 1815–1859* (Chicago, 1960).

7. Starr, "The Old and the New Phrenology," p. 743; William A. Stevenson, "Physiological Significance of Vital Force," *PSM* 24 (April 1884): 769; William A. Hammond, *A Treatise on Insanity in Its Medical Relations* (New York, 1883), p. 13. The relation of body and brain to mind has remained unresolvable for neurophysiologists. In this essay we

have tried to reconstruct the most widely held position in a period in which materialism about brain function was clearly in the ascendancy. E. L. Youmans wrote that the "essence" of mind and matter and "the nature of their union" would forever remain a "mystery," but it was to be the task of the scientist to resolve both systems down to their "simplest elements," which to Youmans meant more localization studies. Writing in 1879, when he was deeply involved in physiological psychology, William James was contemptuous of consciousness as the "unscientific half of existence," unopen to experimental testing, and somehow "inert, uninfluential," and contemptible, although he was later equally contemptuous of equating brain activity with phosphorus excretion. With less venom, Henry Maudsley suggested that scientists might never "bridge the gap" between nerve molecules and consciousness, but should more modestly be engaged in ascertaining "uniformities of [molecular] sequence," leaving the mysterious union alone. Joseph Le-Conte, an older scientific generalist, a "naturalist," who was of a more religious turn of mind than most physiologists, was the leading American proponent of "correspondence," psychology and physiology traveling along separate but parallel series. Like other neurophysiologists, he felt that physiology was "the simpler and more fundamental science," the field open to investigation. Yet unlike other materialist physiologists, he felt that consciousness, though derived from material force, represented "a very distinct form of force," and it could never be dismissed. E. L. Youmans, "Editor's Table: The Relation of Body and Mind," pp. 112–13; William James, "Are We Automata?" *Mind* 4 (January 1879): 1, 3; William James, *Psychology: Briefer Course* (1899) (New York, 1962), pp. 148–49; Henry Maudsley, *Body and Mind* (New York, 1875), pp. 105–6; Joseph LeConte, "Instinct and Intelligence," *PSM* 12 (October 1878): 663–64; E. L. Youmans, "Sketch of Joseph LeConte," *PSM* 12 (January 1878): 358–61. We wish to emphasize the many overlappings of physiological, psychological, and moral categories which characterized almost all neurologists as well as the more popular advisors. For an excellent analysis of this mind/body overlap, set in the context of the ideas of the American neurologist who most nearly freed himself from this confusion of categories, see H. Tristam Englehardt, Jr., "John Hughlings Jackson and the Mind-Body Relation," *BHM* 49 (Summer 1975): 137–49. Physiologists are still trapped, as are many psychologists, on the horns of this duality. See, for example, Wilder Penfield, *The Mystery of the Mind* (Princeton, 1975).

8. Edward C. Spitzka, *Insanity: Its Classification, Diagnosis and Treatment* (New York, 1883), p. 15; Thomas Huxley and W. J. Youmans, *The Elements of Physiology and Hygiene: A Textbook for Educational Institutions*

(New York, 1876), p. 431; Henry Maudsley, *Body and Mind,* p. 40; H. M. Bannister, "Emotional Insanity in Its Medico-Legal Relations," *JNMD* 7 (January 1880): 83–84.

9. Hammond, *A Treatise on Insanity,* p. vii.

10. Ibid., p. v.

11. B. W. Richardson, *The Diseases of Modern Life,* (New York, 1876), pp. 124–64; Richardson, "Induced Disease from the Influence of thePassions,"*PSM* 8 (November 1875): 61, 66. Two useful brief analyses of nineteenth-century mental illness are Charles A. Rosenberg, *The Trial of the Assassin Guiteau: Psychiatry and Law in the Gilded Age* (Chicago, 1963), pp. 58–64, and Gerald N. Grob, "Mental Illness, Indigency and Welfare: The Mental Hospital in Nineteenth-Century America," in Tamara K. Hareven, ed., *Anonymous Americans: Explorations in Nineteenth-Century Social History* (Englewood Cliffs, N.J., 1971), pp. 250–79.

12. Dain, *Concepts of Insanity,* p. 74; Eric T. Carlson and Norman Dain, "The Meaning of Moral Insanity," *BHM* 36 (March 1962): 130–40. Also see Rosenberg, *Guiteau,* pp. 68–70.

Dain, writing with Eric T. Carlson, stresses that by 1870, "degeneracy" had superseded the earlier use of moral insanity, and that later in the century degeneracy was in turn replaced by "evolutionism," and then in the twentieth century, by "personality disorders" as an explanatory device for antisocial behavior. They emphasize that the symptoms of disorder remain the same although the term *moral insanity* eventually died. In our reading we have found that the term and concept of *moral insanity* overlapped chronologically with these other definitions, and in popular usage remained dominant until the end of the nineteenth century.

13. George M. Beard, *Our Home Physician* (New York, 1870), p. 672; Beard, "The Case of Guiteau—A Psychological Study," *JNMD* 9 (January 1882): 102. Also see W. W. Hall, *The Guide-Board to Health, Peace and Competence* (Springfield, Mass., 1869), pp. 224–26; "Insanity by One Who Has Been Insane," *PSM* 23 (September 1883): 630.

14. Gerald N. Grob, "Mental Illness," and *The State and the Mentally Ill: A History of the Worcester State Hospital in Massachusetts, 1830–1920* (Chapel Hill, N.C., 1966). There is an almost cyclical quality in the belief in the cure of the severely mentally ill. The perfectionist strain in the 1960s, which included the Laingian denial of the very concept of insanity, is currently losing fashion to a perhaps equally modish despair. Somatic pessimism, it must be emphasized, did not always imply self-righteous repudiation of the needs of the insane. It could be linked with a self-consciously enlightened view that whatever the prospects for cure, all the insane should be treated decently. For example, C. Eugene Riggs

argued in 1893 that an insane person was still a person, his individuality was to be respected, and his environment to be made to approximate that of ordinary people. Riggs also felt that it was the duty of the state to see that "all people have the opportunity to be made whole." "An Outline in the Progress in the Care and Handling of the Insane," *JNMD* 20 (September 1893): 620–21. Grob also points out that in the 1890s, there was a trend in psychiatry away from somatic pessimism and toward renewed interest in the psychological (*The State and the Mentally Ill*, p. 268).

15. George M. Beard, *American Nervousness* (New York, 1881), pp. 16–17; Charles E. Rosenberg, "The Place of George M. Beard in Nineteenth-Century Psychiatry," (1962), as revised in Charles E. Rosenberg, *No Other Gods: On Science and American Social Thought* (Baltimore, 1976), pp. 98–108. Two more general essays are John S. Haller, Jr., "Neurasthenia: Medical Profession and Urban 'Blahs,' " *New York State Journal of Medicine* 70 (October 1970): 2489–93; Barbara Sicherman, "The Uses of a Diagnosis; Doctors, Patients, and Neurasthenia," *JHM* 32 (January 1977): 33–54.

16. S. Weir Mitchell, *Doctor and Patient* (Philadelphia, 1888); *Fat and Blood: An Essay on the Treatment of Certain Forms of Neurasthenia and Hysteria* (Philadelphia, 1877); *Lectures on Diseases of the Nervous System, Especially in Women* (Philadelphia, 1881); *Wear and Tear, or Hints for the Overworked* (Philadelphia, 1871). Two useful studies are by Ernest Earnest, *S. Weir Mitchell, Novelist and Physician* (Philadelphia, 1950), and David M. Rein, *S. Weir Mitchell as Psychiatric Novelist* (New York, 1952). Charlotte Perkins Gilman, who had undergone Mitchell's rest cure, later bitterly attacked it as demeaning and infantalizing, in her celebrated short story "The Yellow Wall-Paper" (1891), reprinted in Gail Parker, *The Oven-Birds: American Women on Womanhood* (Garden City, N.Y., 1972), pp. 317–34. Mitchell's techniques were typical, not unique. For similar late nineteenth-century therapies, see, for example, J. Leonard Corning, *Brain Exhaustion* (New York, 1884); *Brain Rest* (New York, 1885); Hammond, *Treatise on Insanity*, pp. 174, 315–16; M. L. Holbrook, *Hygiene of the Brain and Nerves, and the Cure of Nervousness* (New York, 1878)

17. Burt G. Wilder, *What Young People Should Know* (Boston, 1875), pp. 145–47.

18. Leslie Keeley, *The Morphine Eater; or, From Bondage to Freedom* (Dwight, Ill., 1881), p. 20; Beard, *American Nervousness*, p. vi.

19. Corning, *Brain Exhaustion*, pp. 134, 136.

20. J. S. Jewell, "Introductory," *JNMD* 1 (January 1874): 70–71. Also see Holbrook, *Hygiene of the Brain*, p. 52.

21. Beard, *American Nervousness,* p. 120; Huxley and Youmans, *Elements of Physiology and Hygiene,* p. 444.

22. The best contemporary account of late nineteenth-century drug abuse was Harry T. Kane, *Drugs That Enslave: The Opium, Morphine, Chloral and Hasheesh Habits* (Philadelphia, 1881). For a useful modern account, see John S. Haller, Jr., and Robin M. Haller, *The Physician and Sexuality in Victorian America* (Urbana, Ill., 1974), pp. 271–303. Also see H. Wayne Morgan, ed., *Yesterday's Addicts: American Society and Drug Abuse, 1865–1920* (Norman, Okla., 1974).

23. Nathan Allen, "Physiological Basis of Mental Culture," *PSM* 6 (December 1874): 185. Also see Corning, *Brain Exhaustion,* p. 137; John Duffy, "Mental Strain and 'Over-Pressure' in the Schools: A Nineteenth-Century Viewpoint," *JHM* 23 (January 1963): 63–79.

24. *Scribner's,* 4 (June 1872): 244.

25. Edward H. Clarke, *Sex in Education, or a Fair Chance for the Girls* (Boston, 1873), p. 40; R. P. Loring, "The Therapeutics of Puberty," *AJO* 12 (October 1879): 805–6. We call this the Gerald Ford syndrome.

26. Rebuttals to Clarke included Mary Putnam Jacobi, *The Question of Rest for Women During Menstruation* (New York, 1877); Eliza Bisbee Duffey, *No Sex in Education: or, An Equal Chance for Both Girls and Boys* (Syracuse, 1874); and Julia Ward Howe, ed., *Sex and Education: A Reply to Dr. Clarke's Sex in Education* (Boston, 1874). A good recent treatment of the Clarke controversy is Mary Roth Walsh's "The Quirks of a Woman's Brain," in Ruth Hubbard et al., eds., *Women Look at Biology Looking at Women* (Cambridge, Mass. 1979), pp. 103–25.

27. Robert Farquharson, "Mental Overwork," *PSM* 10 (January 1877): 327; Eliza B. Lyman, *The Coming Woman or the Royal Road to Perfection, A Series of Medical Lectures* (Lansing, Mich., 1880), p. 150; also see Joel D. Steele, *Hygienic Physiology* (New York, 1884), p. 190; George M. Beard, *Eating and Drinking* (New York, 1871), pass.; Beard, *Our Home Physician,* pass.; Beard, *American Nervousness,* pass.

28. Allen, "Physiological Basis of Mental Culture," p. 184.

29. R. V. Pierce, *The People's Common-Sense Medical Adviser* (Buffalo, N.Y., 1889), p. 277; P. J. Higgins, "Study, Physiologically Considered," *PSM* 24 (March 1884): 639–45. We analyze the physical education movement in chapter 7.

30. Horatio C. Wood, *Brain-Work and Over-Work* (Philadelphia, 1880), pp. 93–94; Higgins, "Study—Physiologically Considered," p. 640; Corning, *Brain Rest,* p. 39. Also see Edward H. Clarke, *The Building of a Brain* (Boston, 1874).

31. Beard, *Eating and Drinking,* p. 2; Holbrook, *Hygiene of the Brain,* pp. 41, 44; Beard, *American Nervousness,* p. 322. By contrast with

our mercantilist predecessors, we have all become Keynesians of the brain, assuming that we use but a fraction of our available brain cells and that through a variety of techniques, we could enter and exploit vast new inner territories. Perhaps now that our culture is rediscovering the economics of scarcity, the optimism about brain potential will be muted by renewed interest in mental mercantilism.

32. Holbrook, *Hygiene of the Brain,* p. 45.

33. James Sully, *The Teacher's Handbook of Psychology* (New York, 1897), p. 38; Pierce, *The People's Common-Sense Medical Adviser,* pp. 124–25; J. S. Jewell, "Influence of Our Present Civilization in the Production of Nervous and Mental Disease," *JNMD* 8 (January 1881): 3–5.

Making Sense of Sex

Parts of this and the subsequent chapter appeared, in different form, in *The Journal of Sex Research* 17 (August 1981).

1. Charles E. Rosenberg, "Science, Society, and Social Thought" (1966), as revised in Charles E. Rosenberg, *No Other Gods, On Science and American Social Thought* (Baltimore, 1976), p. 5. For the mercantilist metaphor to which we have referred in this paragraph, see William A. Hammond, *Sexual Impotence in the Male* (New York, 1883), p. 126; John H. Kellogg, *Man the Masterpiece* (Battle Creek, Mich., 1892), p. 441; George L. Austin, *Perils of American Women, or a Doctor's Talk with Maiden, Wife, and Mother* (Boston, 1883), p. 88; Joseph W. Howe, *Excessive Venery, Masturbation and Continence* (New York, 1889), pp. 76–77; also see Joel D. Steele, *Hygienic Physiology* (New York, 1884), p. 2; Elizabeth Blackwell, *The Human Element in Sex,* rev. ed. (London, 1894), p. 29; S. Pancoast, *Boyhood's Perils and Manhood's Curse* (Philadelphia, 1873), p. 31. The analogy between sexual and capitalist savings has been advanced most fully in Peter T. Cominos, "Late Victorian Respectability and the Social System," *International Review of Social History* 8 (1963): 19–48; 216–50.

2. Sigmund Freud, *Civilization and Its Discontents,* ed. and trans. James Strachey (New York, 1962), p. 51; Paul Robinson, *The Modernization of Sex* (New York, 1976), p. 61. For a discussion of culture specific impulse control, see Hanna Papanek, "Purdah: Separate Worlds and Symbolic Shelter," *Comparative Studies in Society and History* 15 (June 1973): 316. Notions of plenty coexisted with these scarcity suppositions, as in Henry Ward Beecher's sermons of the 1850s, "The Fullness of God" and "Grace Abounding," in which he declared that "In every part of life God has fruit ready to drop into your lap," but in economic and social *metaphors,* this was a minority assumption until the very end of the

nineteenth century. Daniel T. Rodgers, *The Work Ethic in Industrial America 1850–1920* (Chicago, 1978), pp. 97–99.

3. Henry Maudsley, *Body and Will: Metaphysical, Physiological and Pathological Aspects* (New York, 1884), p. 167.

4. For late twentieth-century struggles to make sense of American Victorian sexual ideology and mores, see Charles E. Rosenberg, "Sexuality, Class and Role in Nineteenth Century America" (1973), as revised in *No Other Gods,* pp. 71–88; Carroll Smith-Rosenberg, "The Hysterical Woman: Sex Roles and Role Conflict in Nineteenth Century America," *Social Research* 39 (Winter 1972): 652–78; Carroll Smith-Rosenberg and Charles E. Rosenberg, "The Female Animal: Medical and Biological Views of the Woman and Her Role in Nineteenth-Century America" (1973), as revised in *No Other Gods,* pp. 54–70; Carroll Smith-Rosenberg, "Sex as Symbol in Victorian Purity: An Ethnohistorical Analysis of Jacksonian America," *American Journal of Sociology* 84, Supplement (1978); S212–47. Carl Degler, "What Ought To Be and What Was: Women's Sexuality in the Nineteenth Century," *American Historical Review* 79 (December 1974): 1467–90; Michael Bliss, "Pure Books on Avoided Subjects: Pre-Freudian Sexual Ideals in Canada," *Historical Papers* (Canadian Historical Association, 1970); Linda Gordon, *Woman's Body, Woman's Right; a Social History of Birth Control in America* (New York, 1976); David M. Kennedy, *Birth Control in America: The Career of Margaret Sanger* (New Haven, 1970); Nathan G. Hale, Jr., *Freud and the Americans: The Beginnings of Psychoanalysis in the United States, 1876–1917* (New York, 1971); John S. Haller, Jr., and Robin M. Haller, *The Physician and Sexuality in Victorian America* (Urbana, Ill., 1974); Ronald G. Walters, *Primers for Prudery: Sexual Advice to Victorian America* (Englewood Cliffs, N.J., 1974); David J. Pivar, *Purity Crusade: Sexual Morality and Social Control, 1868–1900* (Westport, Conn., 1974); G. J. Barker-Benfield, *The Horrors of the Half-Known Life: Male Attitudes Toward Women and Sexuality in Nineteenth-Century America* (New York, 1975), which we reviewed at length in *Reviews in American History* 4 (December 1976): 558–64; Hal Sears, *The Sex Radicals: Free Love in High Victorian America* (Lawrence, Kans., 1977); Nancy F. Cott, "Passionlessness: An Interpretation of Victorian Sexual Ideology, 1790–1850," *Signs* 4 (Winter 1978): 219–30; Carl Degler, *At Odds, Women and the Family in America from the Revolution to the Present* (New York, 1980), esp. chaps. 7–12.

5. Quoted in Hugh Hodge, *Foeticide or Criminal Abortion* (Philadelphia, 1869), pp. 6–8. Mary Ryan points out that after 1830 neither the church nor the family retained its formal control over the individual's private sexual behavior. Until this point in Utica, New York, for example, Protestant churches empowered their elders to examine and chastise

their members on the subject of their fornication and adultery. After the early 1830s, following ecclesiastical debates on this issue, local churches ceased using this method of enforcing sexual morality, while increasing religious diversity prevented any one church from claiming to speak for all individuals' sexual codes in the town. Mary P. Ryan, "The Power of Women's Networks: A Case Study of Female Moral Reform in Antebellum America," *Feminist Studies* 5 (Spring 1979): 71–72. Degler summarizes recent scholarship concerning the decline in family size in *At Odds,* chap. 8.

6. Anonymous, *The Truth About Love* (New York, 1872), p. 31; Linda Gordon, *Woman's Body,* p. 98.

7. James C. Mohr, *Abortion in America; The Origins and Evolution of National Policy, 1800–1900* (New York, 1978), pp. 102, 145, 240.

8. Hodge, *Foeticide,* pp. 32–33.

9. William Goodell, *Lessons in Gynecology* (Philadelphia, 1879), p. 374.

10. The central content of the law prohibited interstate distribution of obscene literature through the mails, but the law was interpreted broadly enough to include contraceptive information which was defined as obscene by federal authorities. This law was buttressed by many state antiobscenity and anticontraceptive laws. One advisor, Edward Bliss Foote, was prosecuted in 1876 for circulating a birth control manual. Carol Flora Brooks, "The Early History of the Anti-Contraceptive Laws in Massachusetts and Connecticut," *American Quarterly* 18 (Spring 1966): 9; also see Norman E. Himes, *Medical History of Contraception* (New York, 1970), pp. 260–85; Gordon, *Woman's Body,* pp. 47–71; Ernest C. Helm, "The Prevention of Contraception," *Medical and Surgical Reporter* 59 (November 1888): 645; "The Prevention of Conception: From the Proceedings of the Detroit Medical Association," *Cincinnati Medical News* 19 (1890): 303–8, quoted in John Paull Harper, "Be Fruitful and Multiply: Origins of Legal Restrictions on Planned Parenthood in Nineteenth-Century America," in Carol Berkin and Mary Beth Norton, eds., *Women of America: A History* (Boston, 1979), p. 268.

11. Andrew Nebinger, *Criminal Abortion: Its Extent and Prevention* (Philadelphia, 1870), p. 9; Dr. Davendorf is quoted in Harper, "Be Fruitful and Multiply," p. 268.

12. Nathan Allen, "The Law of Human Increase," *PSM* 22 (November 1882): 42.

13. Nebinger, *Criminal Abortion,* pp. 17, 21–24; Hodge, *Foeticide,* p. 33; James C. Reed, *Private Vice to Public Virtue, Birth Control in America, 1830 to the Present* (New York, 1978), p. 17.

14. Anonymous, *The Truth About Love,* p. 23.

15. William A. Hammond, *Sexual Impotence in the Male,* p. 26.

16. Cott, "Passionlessness," pp. 219–36; Hodge, *Foeticide,* p. 34.

17. Hodge, *Foeticide,* p. 33; Nebinger, *Criminal Abortion,* p. 19; Reed, *Private Vice to Public Virtue,* p. x.

18. Sears, *Sex Radicals,* p. 22.

19. Gordon, *Woman's Body,* pp. 95–115; Horatio R. Storer, *Is It I? A Book for Every Man* (Boston, 1868), p. 117; also see Eliza Barton Lyman, *The Coming Woman, or the Royal Road to Perfection: A Series of Medical Lectures* (Lansing, Mich., 1880), pp. 207, 255; Russell T. Trall, *Sexual Physiology: A Scientific and Popular Exposition of the Fundamental Problems in Sociology,* 13th ed. (New York, 1872), p. 244.

20. Gordon, *Woman's Body,* pp. 95–96; Reed, *Private Vice to Public Virtue,* p. 25; Lois W. Banner, *Elizabeth Cady Stanton. A Radical for Women's Rights* (Boston, 1980), pp. 84, 114–15, 124; Sears, *Sex Radicals,* p. 22; also see Daniel Scott Smith, "Family Limitation, Sexual Control and Domestic Feminism," in Mary Hartman and Lois Banner, eds., *Clio's Consciousness Raised: New Perspectives on the History of Women* (New York, 1974).

21. John Modell, Frank F. Furstenberg, Jr., and Theodore Hershberg, "Social Change and Transitions to Adulthood in Historical Perspective," in Michael Gordon, ed., *The American Family in Social-Historical Perspective,* 2d ed. (New York, 1978), pp. 203, 214.

22. R. P. Neuman, "Masturbation, Madness and the Modern Concepts of Childhood and Adolescence," *JSH* 8 (Spring 1975): 1–27; J. Hamilton Ayres, *Every Man His Own Doctor: A Family Medical Advisor* (New York, 1879), p. 247.

23. Henry G. Hanchett, *Sexual Health,* 2d ed. (New York, 1889), p. 62. Carroll Smith-Rosenberg argues that in the Jacksonian era, adolescent male masturbation symbolized the potential ungovernability of the most rootless and troublesome group in American society ("Sex as Symbol," pp. S219–20).

24. Hammond, *Sexual Impotence in the Male,* pp. 110–11.

25. Daniel Scott Smith, "The Dating of the American Sexual Revolution: Evidence and Interpretation," in Gordon, ed., *The American Family,* p. 434; Harper, "Be Fruitful and Multiply," p. 260.

26. Sears, *Sex Radicals,* pp. 27, 81–82, 271–72.

The Rule of Moderation in Sexual Ideology

1. Henry Maudsley, *Body and Will: Metaphysical, Physiological and Pathological Aspects* (New York, 1884), p. 167.

2. Elizabeth Blackwell, *The Human Element in Sex,* rev. ed. (London, 1894), p. 29.

3. R. V. Pierce, *The People's Common Sense Medical Adviser,* 21st ed. (Buffalo, 1889), p. 209.

4. Pierce, *Medical Adviser,* p. 192; Elizabeth Blackwell, *The Moral Education of the Young in Relation to Sex* (1879), in *Essays in Medical Sociology,* 2 vols. (London, 1902), 1: 258; Rev. George W. Hudson, *The Marriage Guide for Young Men, A Manual of Courtship and Marriage* (Ellsworth, Me., 1883), pp. 96–97.

5. Joseph W. Howe, *Excessive Venery, Masturbation and Continence* (New York, 1889), pp. 183–200; W. R. D. Blackwell, "The Prevention of Conception," *Medical and Surgical Reporter* 59 (September 1888): 396; William A. Hammond, *Sexual Impotence in the Male* (New York, 1883), p. 25; and George H. Napheys, *The Transmission of Life: Counsels on the Nature and Hygiene of the Masculine Function,* 14th ed. (Philadelphia, 1877), p. 250, who recommended continence as a limited therapeutic tool for sexual disorders rather than as a panacea.

6. J. T. Kent, *Sexual Neuroses* (St. Louis, 1879), p. 21.

7. Russell T. Trall, *Sexual Physiology: A Scientific and Popular Exposition of the Fundamental Propositions in Sociology,* 13th ed. (New York, 1872), pp. 68–69; Charles Rosenberg has suggested that women who believed orgasm was necessary to impregnation may have suppressed sexual excitement as a means of birth control: (1973) "Sexuality, Class and Role in Nineteenth-Century America," in *No Other Gods, On Science and American Social Thought* (Baltimore, 1976), p. 76.

8. Henry G. Hanchett, *Sexual Health,* 2d ed. (New York, 1889), p. 62.

9. Horatio R. Storer, *Is It I? A Book for Every Man* (Boston, 1868), p. 117; George L. Austin, *Perils of American Women, or a Doctor's Talk with Maiden, Wife and Mother* (Boston, 1883), p. 88; Blackwell, *The Moral Education of the Young,* p. 258; Trall, *Sexual Physiology,* pp. 241–42; Henry Guernsey, *Plain Talk on Avoided Subjects* (Philadelphia, 1882), p. 103.

10. J. R. Black, *The Ten Laws of Health or How Disease Is Produced and Can Be Prevented* (Philadelphia, 1885), p. 233; also see Eliza Barton Lyman, *The Coming Woman, or the Royal Road to Perfection: A Series of Medical Lectures* (Lansing, Mich., 1880), p. 242; Nicholas E. Boyd, ed., *Plain Sober Talk to the Studious About Our Sexual Nature* (Washington, D.C., 1875), p. 4; John Cowan, *The Science of a New Life* (New York, 1871), pass.; Howe, *Excessive Venery,* pp. 95–96; Dio Lewis, *Chastity or Our Secret Sins* (New York, 1890), pp. 58, 84–85.

11. Boyd, *Sober Talk*, pp. 5–6; also see Burt G. Wilder, *What Young People Should Know: The Reproductive Organs in Man and the Lower Animals* (Boston, 1875), p. 147; Lewis, *Chastity,* pass.; John H. Kellogg, *Plain Facts For Old and Young* (Burlington, Iowa, 1889), p. 162; Austin, *Perils of American Women,* p. 89.

12. Charles Rosenberg, "Sexuality, Class and Role," pp. 71–88; Philip Greven, *The Protestant Temperament: Patterns of Child-Bearing, Religious Experience and the Self in Early America* (New York, 1977).

13. Trall, *Sexual Physiology,* pp. 202, 229, 266; see also John H. Dye, *Painless Childbirth; or Healthy Mothers and Healthy Children,* 2d ed. (Silver Creek, N.Y. 1882), p. 14. *Pornotopia* is explored in Stephen Marcus, *The Other Victorians: A Study of Sexuality and Pornography in Mid-Nineteenth-Century England* (New York, 1966).

14. Dye, *Painless Childbirth,* p. 17; also see B. W. Richardson, "Induced Disease from the Influence of the Passions," *PSM* 8 (November 1875): 60–65; Pierce, *Medical Adviser,* p. 204.

15. Lyman, *The Coming Woman,* pp. 218–19; also see Pierce, *Medical Adviser,* p. 291; William M. Capp, *The Daughter, Her Health, Education, and Wedlock* (Philadelphia, 1891), p. 71; Hudson, *Marriage Guide,* p. 245; William James, *Psychology: Briefer Course* (New York, 1962), pp. 117–18.

16. Blackwell, *The Human Element in Sex,* pp. 11–12.

17. Cowan, *Science of a New Life,* p. 99.

18. Review of C. A. Greene's *Build Well: Plain Truths Relating to the Obligations of Marriage,* in *PSM* 44 (February 1894): 557; Augustus K. Gardner, *Conjugal Sins: Against the Laws of Life and Health and Their Effects upon the Father, Mother, and Child* (New York, 1870), p. 80; Alice B. Stockham, *Tokology: A Book for Every Woman* (Chicago, 1885), p. 140; George M. Beard, *Sexual Neurasthenia* (New York, 1886), p. 103; Hal Sears, *The Sex Radicals* (Lawrence, Kans., 1977), p. 272; also see Kellogg, *Plain Facts,* p. 110; Wilder, *Young People,* p. 147; Hammond, *Sexual Impotence,* p. 130; Trall, *Sexual Physiology,* pp. 229–34; Hudson, *Marriage Guide,* pp. 243–44.

19. Trall, *Sexual Physiology,* p. 243.

20. Austin, *Perils of American Women,* p. 89; Napheys, *Transmission of Life,* p. 29; Dye, *Painless Childbirth,* p. 14; Hudson, *Marriage Guide,* p. 97; Pierce, *Medical Adviser,* p. 291; Eli F. Brown, *Sex and Life: The Physiology and Hygiene of the Sexual Organization* (Chicago, 1891), p. 52.

21. Elaine Tyler May writes that in a sample of divorce cases of the 1880s, those involving sexual conflicts almost always revolved around the wife's charge of her husband's abusive conduct, by which was meant nightly intercourse, even during menstruation, without regard for the wife's health or wishes. May notes that such sexual complaints gener-

ally convinced the court. See her *Great Expectations, Marriage and Divorce in Post-Victorian America* (Chicago, 1980), pp. 33, 36.

22. Cowan, *Science of a New Life,* pp. 170, 174. In an odd way, Cowan is like a William Morris of sexuality, arguing for the well-crafted, old-fashioned artifact in the place of countless, shabby, machine-produced objects.

23. Storer, *Is It I?,* p. 117; Lyman, *The Coming Woman,* pp. 207, 255; Trall, *Sexual Physiology,* p. 244; and on voluntary motherhood, see Linda Gordon, *Woman's Body, Woman's Right: A Social History of Birth Control in America* (New York, 1976), pp. 95–115.

24. Edward Bliss Foote, *Medical Common Sense and Plain Home Talk* (New York, 1883), p. 872. Here, it is interesting to note, it was the woman, not the man, whose sexual fluids were in short supply.

25. Beard, *Sexual Neurasthenia,* p. 200.

26. Kellogg, *Plain Facts,* pp. 110–11.

27. Hammond, *Sexual Impotence,* pp. 94, 190–91.

28. Austin, *Perils of American Women,* p. 36.

29. Ibid., pp. 92–93, 95; Boyd, *Sober Talk,* p. 6; Cowan, *Science of a New Life,* p. 194; Dye, *Painless Childbirth,* pp. 71–72.

30. Gardner, *Conjugal Sins,* pp. 150–51; also see George H. Napheys, *The Physical Life of Women* (Philadelphia, 1870), p. 303.

31. Prudence B. Saur, *Maternity: A Book for Every Wife and Mother* (Chicago, 1891), p. 55. In *The Physical Life of Women,* p. 301, Napheys urges temperance rather than continence during this critical time.

32. Austin, *Perils of American Women,* p. 87.

33. Napheys, *Transmission of Life,* p. 36; Gardner, *Conjugal Sins,* pp. 173–74; also see Hammond, *Sexual Impotence,* pp. 132–33.

34. Vern L. Bullough and Martha Voght, "Homosexuality and Its Confusion with the 'Secret Sin' in Pre-Freudian America," *JHM* 28 (April 1973): 143–55; Hammond, *Sexual Impotence,* p. 26; also see A. C. McClanahan, "An Investigation into the Effects of Masturbation," *New York Medical Journal* 66 (1897): 502, in which masturbation is characterized as "selfish, solitary," completely lacking in anything "akin to love or sympathy"; also see Arthur N. Gilbert, "Doctor, Patient and Onanist Diseases in the Nineteenth Century," *JHM* 30 (1975): 224–25.

35. William Hammond, *Sexual Impotence in the Male and Female* (Detroit, 1887), pp. 302–3; Napheys, *The Physical Life of Women,* p. 35; Blackwell, *The Human Element in Sex,* pp. 40–41. Horatio Storer thought masturbation much more immoral than legalized prostitution, which he favored (*Is It I?,* p. 48).

36. Austin, *Perils of American Women,* p. 54; Hammond, *Sexual Impotence,* p. 92; Beard, *Sexual Neurasthenia,* p. 200; Howe, *Excessive Venery,*

pp. 76–77; also see Joel D. Steele, *Hygienic Physiology* (New York, 1884), p. 2; Blackwell, *The Human Element in Sex,* p. 29; S. Pancoast, *Boyhood's Perils and Manhood's Curse* (Philadelphia, 1873), p. 31.

37. Hammond, *Sexual Impotence,* p. 126; also see Storer, *Is It I?,* p. 123; Martin L. Holbrook, *Hygiene of the Brain and Nerves and the Cure of Nervousness* (New York, 1878), p. 109.

38. Pierce warned also of the puny offspring of chronic masturbators in *Medical Adviser,* p. 816; see also Hammond, *Sexual Impotence in the Male and Female,* p. 302.

39. George M. Beard, *Our Home Physician* (New York, 1870), pp. 818–20.

40. William T. Belfield, *Diseases of the Urinary and Male Sexual Organs* (New York, 1884).

41. Hammond, *Sexual Impotence in the Male,* pp. 82–84. For an analysis of precisely this late-Victorian configuration, see Sigmund Freud, "On the Universal Tendency to Debasement in the Sphere of Love," *Standard Edition* (London, 1957), 11:177–90; and for a mid-Victorian variation on the theme, see Michael Fellman, "Sexual Longing in Richard Henry Dana, Jr.'s American Victorian Diary," *Canadian Review of American Studies* 3 (Fall 1972): 96–105.

42. *Medical and Surgical Reporter,* 59 (September 1888): 342.

43. Kent, *Sexual Neuroses,* p. 21.

44. William A. Hammond, *Sexual Impotence in the Male and Female,* pp. 300–301.

45. Dye, *Painless Childbirth,* p. 16; Hammond, *Sexual Impotence in the Male and Female,* p. 299; Stockham, *Tokology,* p. 140; Hanchett, *Sexual Health,* p. 66. Eliza B. Duffey thought that writers such as Hanchett were selfishly oblivious to the effects of sexual intercourse on women. See *The Relations of the Sexes* (New York, 1889), p. 238.

The Primacy of the Will

An earlier version of this chapter appeared in *Historical Reflections* 4 (Summer 1977): 27–44.

1. William B. Carpenter, "The Unconscious Action of the Brain," *PSM* 1 (September 1872): 560. For Carpenter's place in neurophysiology, see Robert M. Young, *Brain and Adaptation in the Nineteenth Century: Cerebral Localization and its Biological Context from Gall to Ferrier* (Oxford, 1970), pp. 210–20.

2. One widely read text which illustrates this mixing of methods is James Sully, *The Human Mind,* 2 vols., (New York, 1893), and his

popularization for teachers, *Outlines of Psychology* (New York, 1883), esp. pp. 21–26.

3. Carpenter, *The Principles of Mental Physiology* (New York, 1874), pp. 108–9, emphasis added; also see Henry Maudsley, *Body and Will: Metaphysical, Physiological and Pathological Aspects* (New York, 1884), p. 167; William A. Hammond, *A Treatise on Insanity in Its Medical Relations* (New York, 1883), p. 27.

4. William James, "Brute and Human Intellect," *Journal of Speculative Philosophy* 12 (July 1878): 246; Maudsley, *Body and Will*, p. 109.

5. J. Leonard Corning, *Brain Exhaustion* (New York, 1884), p. 50; also Horatio C. Wood, *Brain-Work and Over-Work* (Philadelphia, 1880), p. 68; and Alexander Bain, *The Emotions and the Will*, 3d ed. (New York, 1876). A phrenologist of the older school arrived at the same conclusions: Nelson Sizer, *Forty Years in Phrenology* (New York, 1891), p. 114.

6. Eliza B. Lyman, *The Coming Woman, or the Royal Road to Perfection: A Series of Medical Lectures* (Lansing, Mich., 1880), p. 196.

7. R. L. Dugdale, *The Jukes: A Study in Crime, Pauperism, Disease, and Heredity*, 4th ed. (New York, 1877), p. 43.

8. Carpenter, *The Principles of Mental Physiology*, p. 475.

9. R. V. Pierce, *The People's Common-Sense Medical Adviser*, 21st ed. (Buffalo, 1889), p. 208; also see S. Weir Mitchell, *Doctor and Patient* (Philadelphia, 1888), p. 13.

10. Pierce, *Common-Sense Medical Adviser*, p. 707: also George L. Austin, *Perils of American Women, or A Doctor's Talk with Maiden, Wife, and Mother* (Boston, 1882), p. 185.

11. Horatio Robinson Storer, *Insanity in Women* (Boston, 1871), p. 78.

12. Mitchell, *Doctor and Patient*, pp. 83–84.

13. H. Hughes Bennett, "Hygiene in the Higher Education of Women," *PSM* 16 (February 1880): 522.

14. M. A. Hardaker, "Science and The Woman Question," *PSM* 20 (March 1882): 578. This last point, which was clearly related to the contemporary invidious distinctions drawn between races, was by the 1880s under severe attack. For example, see Miss Nina Morais, "A Reply to Miss Hardaker on the Woman Question," *PSM* 21 (May 1882): 70–78; Joseph Simms, "Human Brain Weights," *PSM* 31 (July 1887): 358–59.

15. S. Weir Mitchell to Mrs. A. G. Mason, November 22, 1912, quoted in David M. Rein, *S. Weir Mitchell as a Psychiatric Novelist* (New York, 1952), p. 52.

16. Austin, *Perils of American Women*, p. 150.

17. Ireneus P. Davis, *Hygiene For Girls* (New York, 1883), p. 114.

18. Frederic R. Marvin, *The Philosophy of Spiritualism and the Pathology and Treatment of Mediomania: Two Lectures* (New York, 1874), p. 47. Here the causal sequence is wonderfully extended: tilted womb to hysteria to radicalism. For a more restrained treatment, see Alex J. C. Skene, "The Relation of the Ovaries to the Brain and Nervous System," *AJO* 14 (January 1881): 54–77.

19. Mitchell, *Doctor and Patient*, p. 138. Parallel statements can be found in Austin, *Perils of American Women*, p. 188; Lyman, *The Coming Woman*, p. 342; Skene, "Relation of the Ovaries," pp. 59–60. Also see Carroll Smith-Rosenberg's article "The Hysterical Woman, Sex Roles and Role Conflict in Nineteenth-Century America," *Social Research* 39 (Winter 1972): 652–78.

20. Ely Van de Warker, "The Genesis of Woman," *PSM* 5 (June 1874): 276.

21. Stephen Smith, *Doctor in Medicine: And Other Papers on Professional Subjects* (New York, 1872), p. 107. This argument suggests that uterine disorders as ideological explanations paralleled the uses made of masturbation by many physicians.

22. Russell T. Trall, *The Health and Diseases of Women* (Battle Creek, Mich., 1873), pp. 16, 17, 23–24. Elsewhere, Trall proclaimed women to be the natural equals of men physically, and in stamina and vital resources the superior: *The Mother's Hygienic Hand-Book* (New York, 1874), p. 6. Also see Robert Latou Dickinson, "Bicycling for Women from the Standpoint of the Gynecologist," *AJO* 31 (January 1895): 25.

23. Abba Gould Woolson, *Women in American Society* (Boston, 1873), pp. 193–209. Tight corseting, of course, was as universally condemned by health writers then as were platform shoes in recent days. In a hyperbolic warning, R. T. Trall recounted a tale of "a young lady [who] went to bed without removing her corset, as she wished to grow small. When morning came her friends found her a lifeless corpse." *The Household Manual* (Battle Creek, Mich., 1875), p. 29.

24. Smith, *Doctor in Medicine*, p. 52.

25. Lyman, *The Coming Woman*, p. 301.

26. Elizabeth Cummings, "Education as an Aid to the Health of Women," *PSM* 17 (October 1880): 824.

27. Mitchell, *Doctor and Patient*, p. 131.

28. Mitchell, *Lectures on the Diseases of the Nervous System, Especially in Women* (Philadelphia, 1881), p. 29. Also see Cummings, "Education as an Aid," p. 827, and Frances E. White, "Muscle and Mind," *PSM* 35 (July 1889): 391–92.

29. Maudsley, *Body and Will*, p. 93; Carpenter "The Unconscious Action of the Brain," p. 560.

30. J. H. Kellogg, *Second Book on Physiology and Hygiene* (New York, 1894), p. 223.

31. Hammond, *A Treatise on Insanity,* p. 59; also Edward B. Foote, *Plain Home Talks About the Human System* (New York, 1872), p. 177; Wood, *Brain-Work and Over-Work,* p. 68.

32. William James, "The Laws of Habit," *PSM* 30 (February 1887): 439.

33. Wood, *Brain-Work and Over-Work,* p. 78; also see Joseph Le Conte, "Instinct and Intelligence," *PSM* 7 (October 1875): 661; Elizabeth Blackwell, *The Human Element in Sex,* 2d ed. (London, 1891), pp. 59–62.

34. J. H. Kellogg, *First Book in Physiology and Hygiene* (New York, 1888), p. 133. Interestingly, Kellogg harkened back as well to an older phrenology when he insisted that "the face becomes an index to the character" when the facial "muscles contract habitually a particular way" (*Second Book,* p. 192); E. Vale Blake, "Spontaneous and Imitative Crime," *PSM* 15 (September 1879): 665.

35. Kellogg, *First Book,* p. 139.

36. J. M. W. Kitchen, *Consumption, Its Nature, Causes, Prevention and Cure* (New York, 1885), p. 58.

37. Davis, *Hygiene for Girls,* p. 59; also see Sydney B. Elliott, *Aedeology: A Treatise on Generative Life* (New York, 1892), p. 108; Kellogg, *Second Book,* pp. 223–24, 228–29.

38. Edwin Checkley, *A Natural Method of Physical Training; A Practical Description of the Checkley System of Physiculture* (Brooklyn, 1890), pp. 30, 125.

39. Stephen Freedman, "The Baseball Fad in Chicago, 1865–1870: An Exploration of the Role of Sport in the Nineteenth-Century City," *Journal of Sport History* 5 (Summer 1978): 50.

40. "Dio Lewis," in *American Medical Biographies,* Howard A. Kelly and Walter L. Burrage, eds. (Baltimore, 1920), p. 699; Roberta J. Park, " 'Embodied Selves': The Rise and Development of Concern for Physical Education, Active Games and Recreation for American Women, 1776–1865," *Journal of Sport History* 5 (Summer 1978): 28.

41. William James, *Psychology: Briefer Course* (reprint ed., New York, 1962), pp. 162–63; D. H. Jacques, *How to Grow Handsome* (New York, 1890), pp. xvi, 31.

42. Wood, *Brain-Work and Over-Work,* p. 92.

43. Genevieve Stebbins, *Society Gymnastics and Voice-Culture Adapted from the Delsarte System,* 6th ed. (New York, 1888), p. 7.

44. Carl Betz, *A System of Physical Culture* (Kansas City, Mo., 1887), frontispiece. See also Nils Posse, *The Swedish System of Educational*

Gymnastics (Boston, 1890), p. 3; Mara L. Pratt, *The New Calisthenics: A Manual of Health and Beauty* (Boston, 1889), p. 4; Stebbins, *Society Gymnastics and Voice-Culture,* p. 7.

45. John Boyle O'Reilly, *Ethics of Boxing and Manly Sport* (Boston, 1888), p. xv.

46. Charles W. Emerson, *Physical Culture* (Boston, 1881), p. 33.

47. Edwin Checkley, however, rejected the idea that present modes of life could not naturally yield strong bodies: "It is stating a simple truth to say that a man or woman should get good health and sufficient strength and perfection of form in the ordinary activities of life, if these activities, however meagre, are carried on in obedience to right laws" (*A Natural Method of Physical Training,* p. 18). This release from responsibility for vigorous exercise apparently relieved the minds of many respectable people, judging from the testimonials at the back of Checkley's book.

48. S. M. Barnett, "Barnett's Patent Parlor Gymnasium and Chest Expander for Schools and Families" (New York, 1871), p. 7; also see Joseph C. Hutchinson, *A Treatise on Physiology and Hygiene for Educational Institutions and General Readers* (New York, 1892), p. 36.

49. Richard A. Proctor, "Growth and Decay of Mind," *PSM* 4 (January 1874): 329.

50. Eugene L. Richards, "The Influence of Exercise upon Health," *PSM* 29 (July 1886): 334; also see White, "Muscle and Mind," p. 378; Kellogg, *Second Book,* p. 200.

51. Posse, *Swedish System,* p. 240; William Blaikie, *Sound Bodies for Our Boys and Girls* (New York, 1881), p. iii.

52. William Blaikie, *How to Get Strong and How to Stay So* (New York, 1879), p. 77; Stebbins, *Society Gymnastics,* p. 8; Posse, *Swedish System,* p. 239; also see George M. Beard, *American Nervousness* (New York, 1881), pass.

53. Felix L. Oswald, *Physical Education* (New York, 1882), p. 122; also see Ed. James, *How to Acquire Health, Strength and Muscle,* 3d ed. (New York, 1877), p. 6.

54. Posse, *Swedish System,* p. 2; Alfred Worcester, "Gymnastics," *PSM* 23 (May 1883): 82; William Dick, *Dick's Art of Gymnastics* (New York, 1885), p. 6.

55. Alice Rossi, ed., *The Feminist Papers* (New York, 1974), pp. 114, 105–7, quoted in Park, " 'Embodied Selves,' " p. 14.

56. Ibid., pp. 13–21.

57. Checkley, *A Natural Method of Physical Training,* p. 102.

58. Charlotte Perkins Gilman, *The Living of Charlotte Perkins Gilman: An Autobiography* (New York, 1935), pp. 28–33, 56.

59. James, *How to Acquire Health,* p. 7; for a full discussion of the same manly beau ideal in Victorian England, see Bruce Haley, *The Healthy Body and Victorian Culture* (Cambridge, Mass., 1978).

60. Boston Normal School of Gymnastics, (First) *Annual Catalogue* (Boston, 1892), p. 6.

61. Julian Hawthorne, "The Building of the Muscle," *Harper's Monthly* 69 (August 1884): 384.

62. Richards, "College Athletics," *PSM* 24 (March 1884): 593.

63. Bernarr A. McFadden, *The Virile Powers of Superb Manhood; How Developed, How Lost, How Regained* (New York, 1900), p. 198.

64. James C. Whorton, "The Hygiene of the Wheel: An Episode in Victorian Sanitary Science," *BHM* 52 (Spring 1978): 69, 74.

65. Carpenter, *The Principles of Mental Physiology,* pp. 650–51.

66. Letter in Detroit *Lancet* 8 (1884–85): 251–54, reprinted in H. Wayne Morgan, ed., *Yesterday's Addicts: American Society and Drug Abuse 1865–1920* (Norman, Okla., 1974), pp. 147–52.

67. Davis, *Hygiene for Girls,* pp. 209–10; also see Blackwell's *The Human Element in Sex,* pp. 63–64; J. Mortimer-Granville, *Youth: Its Care and Culture* (New York, 1882), p. 56.

68. Hammond, *A Treatise on Insanity,* p. 210; also see Kellogg, *Plain Facts for Old and Young* (Burlington, Iowa, 1889), p. 296.

69. Ibid., p. 31; also see Beard, "A New Theory of Trance, and Its Bearing on Human Testimony," *JNMD* 4 (January 1877): 5. William James was more open than these others to psychic experiences, as long as solid citizens were doing the experiencing. See James B. Gilbert, *Work Without Salvation: America's Intellectuals and Industrial Alienation 1880–1910* (Baltimore, 1977), p. 201.

70. Carpenter, *The Principles of Mental Physiology,* p. 391; also see Charles E. Rosenberg, *The Trial of the Assassin Guiteau: Psychiatry and Law in the Gilded Age* (Chicago, 1963), p. 58.

71. Sir James Crichton-Browne, "Responsibility in Mental Disease," *PSM* 36 (November 1889): 82–83.

72. Corning, *Brain Exhaustion,* p. 60; also see Blackwell, "The Religion of Health" (1871), in *Essays in Medical Sociology* (London, 1902), 2:217.

73. Maudsley, *Body and Will,* p. 266.

Conclusion

1. This is the general theme of James M. Gilbert, *Work Without Salvation: America's Intellectuals and Industrial Alienation, 1880–1910* (Baltimore, 1977).

2. Paul Boyer, *Urban Masses and Moral Order in America, 1820–1920* (Cambridge, Mass., 1978).

3. Daniel T. Rodgers, *The Work Ethic in Industrial America, 1850–1920* (Chicago, 1978), p. 123.

4. Luther Lee Bernard, "The Transition to an Objective Standard of Social Control," *American Journal of Sociology* 16 (1911): 210, 532–33, quoted in Boyer, *Urban Masses and Moral Order,* p. 231.

5. Lewis Thomas, "Notes of a Biology Watcher: The Health-Care System," *New England Journal of Medicine* 293 (December 1975): 1246. Also see Lewis Thomas, "A Meliorist View of Disease and Dying," *Journal of Medicine and Philosophy* 1 (1976): 212–21. We are much obliged to Dr. Thomas for offprints he sent us of his work.

6. E. D. Pellegrino, "Medicine, History and the Idea of Man," in J. A. Clausen and R. Straus, eds., *Medicine and Society. Annals of the American Academy of Political and Social Sciences* 346 (1963): 9.

7. Five strong studies of nineteenth-century America based on a notion of coercive authority are Michael B. Katz, *The Irony of Early School Reform: Educational Innovation in Mid-Nineteenth Century Massachusetts* (Cambridge, Mass., 1968); David J. Rothman, *The Discovery of the Asylum: Social Order and Disorder in the New Republic* (Boston, 1971); Lawrence J. Friedman, *Inventors of the Promised Land* (New York, 1975); Burton J. Bledstein, *The Culture of Professionalism: The Middle Class and the Development of Higher Education in America* (New York, 1976); Ronald T. Takaki, *Iron Cages: Race and Culture in Nineteenth-Century America* (New York, 1979).

8. Sacvan Bercovitch, *The American Jeremiad* (Madison, Wis., 1979); Donald M. Scott, *From Office to Profession: The New England Ministry, 1750–1850* (Philadelphia, 1978); Kathryn Kish Sklar, *Catharine Beecher: A Study in American Domesticity* (New Haven, 1973); Ann Douglas, *The Feminization of American Culture* (New York, 1977); Gwendolyn Wright, *Moralism and the Modern Home: Domestic Architecture and Cultural Conflict in Chicago, 1873–1913* (Chicago, 1980).

9. An elegant essay which best states this tendency is David P. Hollinger, "Historians and the Discourse of Intellectuals," in John Higham and Paul Conkin, eds., *New Directions in American Intellectual History* (Baltimore, 1979).

10. Two assaults on social history from this general perspective are Elizabeth Fox Genovese and Eugene D. Genovese, "The Political Crisis of Social History: A Marxian Perspective," *JSH* 10 (Winter 1976): 205–20; Tony Judt, "A Clown in Regal Purple: Social History and the Historians," *History Workshop* 7 (Spring 1979): 66–94.

11. The work of Bernard Bailyn and Gordon Wood on the American Revolution and David Brion Davis on the nineteenth century

are the most thoroughly developed analyses of popular political ideology. A good synthesis of ideology and structure is Robert Kelly, *The Cultural Pattern in American Politics: The First Century* (New York, 1979). Two analyses of popular ideology in the crisis of the Civil War era are Michael Fellman, "Rehearsal for the Civil War: Antislavery and Proslavery at the Fighting Point in Kansas, 1854–1856," in Lewis Perry and Michael Fellman, eds., *Antislavery Reconsidered: New Perspectives on the Abolitionists* (Baton Rouge, La., 1979), pp. 287–307; and Eric Foner, *Free Soil, Free Labor, Free Men: The Ideology of the Republican Party Before the Civil War* (New York, 1970).

Bibliography

Books and Articles by the Advisors and Their Contemporaries

Allen, Nathan. "The Law of Human Increase." *PSM* 22 (November 1882).
———. "Physiological Basis of Mental Culture." *PSM* 6 (December 1874).
Austin, George L. *Perils of American Womanhood, or a Doctor's Talk with Maiden, Wife, and Mother.* Boston: Lee and Shepard, 1883.
Ayres, Hamilton. *Every Man His Own Doctor: A Family Medical Adviser.* New York: G. N. Carleton, 1879.

Bain, Alexander. *Mind and Body.* New York: D. Appleton, 1873.
———. *The Emotions and the Will.* 3d. ed. New York: D. Appleton, 1876.
Bannister, H. M. "Emotional Insanity in Its Medico-Legal Relations." *JNMD* 7 (January 1880): 79–98.

Barnett, S. M. *Barnett's Patent Parlor Gymnasium and Chest Expander for Schools and Families.* New York: J. Becker, 1871.

Bayard, Edward. "Homeopathy as a Science." *PSM* 23 (October 1883): 738–41.

Beard, George M. *American Nervousness.* New York: G. P. Putnam, 1881.

———. *Eating and Drinking.* New York: G. P. Putnam, 1871.

———. *Our Home Physician.* New York: E. B. Treat, 1869.

———. *Sexual Neurasthenia.* New York: E. B. Treat, 1884.

———. "A New Theory of Trance, and Its Bearing on Human Testimony." *JNMD* 4 (January 1877): 1–47.

———. "The Case of Guiteau—A Psychological Study." *JNMD* 9 (January 1882): 90–125.

———, and Rockwell, A. D. *On the Medical and Surgical Uses of Electricity.* 8th ed. New York: W. Wood, 1891.

Bennett, H. Hughes. "Hygiene in the Higher Education of Women." *PSM* 16 (February 1880).

Betz, Carl. *A System of Physical Culture.* 3d. ed. Kansas City, Mo.: Kansas City Presse, 1888.

Black, J. R. *The Ten Laws of Health or How Disease Is Produced and Can Be Prevented.* Philadelphia: J. B. Lippincott, 1885.

———. "Removal of Inherited Tendencies to Disease." *PSM* 15 (August 1879).

Blackwell, Elizabeth. *Essays in Medical Sociology.* 2 vols. London: Ernest Bell, 1902.

———. *The Human Element in Sex.* 2d ed. London: J. A. Churchill, 1894.

Blackwell, W. R. D. "The Prevention of Conception." *Medical and Surgical Reporter* 59 (September 1888).

Blaikie, William. *How to Get Strong and How to Stay So.* New York: Harper and Brothers, 1879.

———. *Sound Bodies for Our Boys and Girls.* New York: Harper and Brothers, 1883.

Blake, E. Vale. "Spontaneous and Imitative Crime." *PSM* 15 (September 1879).

Boston Normal School of Gymnastics. (First) *Annual Catalogue.* Boston, 1892.

Boyd, Nicholas E., ed. *Plain Sober Talk to the Studious About Our Sexual Nature.* Washington, D.C.: Polkinghorn, 1875.

Brown, Eli F. *Sex and Life: The Physiology and Hygiene of the Sexual Organization.* Chicago: F. J. Schulte, 1891.

Capp, William M. *The Daughter, Her Health, Education, and Wedlock.* Philadelphia: F. A. Davis, 1891.

176

Carpenter, William B. *The Principles of Mental Physiology.* New York: Appleton, 1874.

———. "The Unconscious Action of the Brain." *PSM* 1 (September 1870).

Census Office, United States Department of the Interior. *Report on the Population of the United States at the Eleventh Census, 1890.* Washington, D.C., 1895.

Checkley, Edwin. *A Natural Method of Physical Training: A Practical Description of the Checkley System of Physiculture.* Brooklyn: W. C. Bryant, 1890.

Clarke, Edward H. *The Building of a Brain.* Boston: J. R. Osgood, 1874.

———. *Sex in Education or a Fair Chance for the Girls.* Boston: J. R. Osgood, 1873.

Corning, J. Leonard. *Brain Exhaustion.* New York: D. Appleton, 1884.

———. *Brain Rest.* New York: G. P. Putnam, 1885.

Cowan, John. *The Science of a New Life.* New York: Cowan and Company, 1871.

Crichton-Browne, Sir James. "Responsibility in Mental Disease." *PSM* 36 (November 1889).

Crothers, T. D. "New Facts in Alcoholic Heredity." *PSM* 34 (February 1889).

Cummings, Elizabeth. "Education as an Aid to the Health of Women." *PSM* 17 (October 1880).

Davis, Ireneus P. *Hygiene for Girls.* New York, 1883.

Dick, William B. *Dick's Art of Gymnastics.* New York: Dick and Fitzgerald, 1885.

Dickinson, Robert Latou. "Bicycling for Women from the Standpoint of the Gynecologist." *AJO* 31 (January 1895): 24–37.

Duffey, Eliza B. *No Sex in Education: or, An Equal Chance for Both Girls and Boys.* Syracuse, 1874.

———. *The Relations of the Sexes.* New York: Wood and Holbrook, 1876.

Dugdale, R. L. *The Jukes: A Study in Crime, Pauperism, Disease and Heredity.* 4th ed. New York: G. P. Putnam, 1877.

Dye, John. *Painless Childbirth; or Healthy Mothers and Healthy Children.* 2d ed. Silver Creek, N.Y.: Local Printing House, 1882.

Editor's Table. "The Practical Study of Mind." *PSM* 20 (February 1882).

Elliott, Sydney B. *Aedeology: A Treatise on Generative Life.* New York, 1892.

Emerson, Charles W. *Physical Culture.* Boston: Emerson College of Oratory Publishing Department, 1881.

Farquharson, Robert. "Mental Overwork." *PSM* 10 (January 1877).

Fiske, John. *Edward Livingston Youmans.* New York: D. Appleton, 1894.

Foote, Edward B., Jr. *Medical Common Sense and Plain Home Talk.* New York: Murray Hill, 1883.

————. *Plain Home Talks About the Human System.* New York: Wells and Coffin, 1872.

Fothergill, J. Milner. "The Mental Aspects of Ordinary Diseases." *PSM* 6 (March 1875).

French, J. M. "Infant Mortality and the Environment." *PSM* 34 (December 1888): 221–29.

Gardner, Augustus K. *Conjugal Sins: Against the Laws of Life and Health and Their Effects upon the Father, Mother, and Child.* New York: J. S. Redfield, 1870.

Gilman, Charlotte Perkins. *The Living of Charlotte Perkins Gilman: An Autobiography.* New York: D. Appleton-Century, 1935.

————. "The Yellow Wall-Paper." Reprinted in Parker, Gail. *The Oven-Birds: American Women on Womanhood.* Garden City, N.Y.: Doubleday, 1972, pp. 317–34.

Goodell, William. *Lessons in Gynecology.* Philadelphia: D. G. Brinton, 1879.

Gradle, Henry. *Bacteria and the Germ Theory of Disease.* Chicago: W. T. Keener, 1883.

Gross, Samuel W., and Gross, A. Haller, eds. *Autobiography of Samuel D. Gross, M.D.* 2 vols. Philadelphia: H. C. Lea, 1887.

Guernsey, A. H., and Davis, Ireneus P. *Health at Home.* New York: D. Appleton, 1884.

Guernsey, Henry N. *Plain Talk on Avoided Subjects.* Philadelphia: F. A. Davis, 1882.

Hall, W. W. *Fun Better Than Physic; or Everybody's Life-Preserver.* Springfield, Mass.: D. E. Fisk, 1871.

————. *The Guide-Board to Health, Peace and Competence; or The Road to Happy Old Age.* Springfield, Mass.: D. E. Fisk, 1869.

————. *Health and Disease as Affected by Constipation.* New York: Hurd and Houghton, 1870.

————. *Health at Home or Hall's Family Doctor.* Springfield, Mass.: D. E. Fisk, 1887.

————. *Health by Good Living.* New York: Hurd and Houghton, 1875.

Hammond, Clement. "The Prolongation of Human Life." *PSM* 34 (November 1888): 92–101.

Hammond, William A. *Sexual Impotence in the Male*. New York: Berming-ham, 1883.

———. *Sexual Impotence in the Male and Female*. Detroit: G. S. Davis, 1887.

———. *A Treatise on Insanity in Its Medical Relations*. New York: D. Apple-ton, 1883.

Hanchett, Henry G. *Sexual Health*. 2d ed. New York: Buercike & Tafel, 1889.

Hardaker, M. A. "Science and the Woman Question." *PSM* 20 (March 1882).

Hawthorne, Julian. "The Building of the Muscle." *Harper's Monthly* 69 (August 1884).

Helm, Ernest C. "The Prevention of Contraception." *Medical and Surgical Reporter* 59 (November 1888): 645.

Higgins, P. J. "Study—Physiologically Considered." *PSM* 24 (March 1884): 639–45.

Hodge, Hugh L. *Foeticide, or Criminal Abortion: A Lecture Introductory to the Course on Obstetrics and Diseases of Women and Children*. Philadelphia: Lindsay and Blakiston, 1869.

Holbrook, Martin Luther. *Hygiene of the Brain and Nerves and the Cure of Nervousness*. New York: M. L. Holbrook, 1878.

Hoppin, Augustus. *A Fashionable Sufferer*. Boston: Houghton Mifflin, 1883.

"How People Become Ill." *Godey's* 97 (March 1878).

Howe, Joseph W. *Excessive Venery, Masturbation and Continence*. New York: E. B. Trent, 1889.

Howe, Julia Ward, ed. *Sex and Education: A Reply to Dr. Clarke's Sex in Education*. Boston: Roberts Brothers, 1874.

Hudson, Rev. George W. *The Marriage Guide for Young Men: A Manual of Courtship and Marriage*. Ellsworth, Me.: The Author, 1883.

Hutchinson, Joseph L. *A Treatise on Physiology and Hygiene for Educational Institutions and General Readers*. New York: Effingham Maynard, 1892.

Huxley, Thomas H., and Youmans, W. J. *The Elements of Physiology and Hygiene: A Textbook for Educational Institutions*. Rev. ed. New York: D. Appleton, 1876.

"Hypocondria." *Godey's* 99 (August 1879).

"Insanity by One Who Has Been Insane." *PSM* 23 (September 1883).

Jacobi, Mary Putnam. *A Pathfinder in Medicine*. New York: G. P. Putnam, 1925.

————. *The Question of Rest for Women During Menstruation.* New York: G. P. Putnam, 1877.

Jacques, D. H. *How to Grow Handsome.* New York: Fowler and Wells, 1890.

James, Ed. *How to Acquire Health, Strength and Muscle.* 3d ed. New York: E. James, 1877.

James, William. *Psychology, Briefer Course* (1899). Reprinted edition. New York: Collier Books, 1962.

————. *Talks to Teachers on Psychology: And to Students on Some of Life's Ideals* (1899). Reprinted edition. New York: W. W. Norton, 1958.

————. "Are We Automata?" *Mind* 4 (January 1879).

————. "Brute and Human Intellect." *Journal of Speculative Philosophy* 12 (July 1878).

————. "The Laws of Habit." *PSM* 30 (February 1887).

Jewell, J. S. "Influence of Our Present Civilization in the Production of Nervous and Mental Disease." *JNMD* 8 (January 1881): 1–24.

————. "Introductory." *JNMD* 1 (January 1874): 70–73.

Kane, Harry. *Drugs that Enslave: The Opium, Morphine, Chloral and Hasheesh Habits.* Philadelphia: P. Blakiston, 1881.

————. "A Hashish House in New York." *Harper's Monthly* 67 (November 1883): 944–49.

Keeley, Leslie E. *The Morphine Eater; or, from Bondage to Freedom.* Dwight, Ill.: C. L. Palmer, 1881.

Kellogg, J. H. *First Book in Physiology and Hygiene.* New York: Harper, 1888.

————. *Man the Masterpiece.* Battle Creek, Mich.: Good Health, 1892.

————. *Plain Facts for Old and Young.* Burlington, Iowa: I. F. Segner, 1889.

————. *Second Book on Physiology and Hygiene.* New York: American Book, 1894.

Kelly, Howard A., and Burrage, Walter L., eds. *American Medical Biographies.* Baltimore: Norman, Remington, 1920.

Kent, J. T. *Sexual Neuroses.* St. Louis: Maynard and Tedford, 1879.

Kitchen, J. M. W. *Consumption, Its Nature, Causes, Prevention and Cure.* New York: G. P. Putnam, 1885.

LeConte, Joseph. "Instinct and Intelligence." *PSM* 12 (October 1878).

Lewis, Dio. *Chastity or Our Secret Sins.* New York: Arno, 1890.

————. *Our Digestion; or My Jolly Friend's Secret.* Philadelphia: G. Maclean, 1872.

————. *Talks About People's Stomachs.* Boston: Fields, Osgood, 1870.

Loring, R. P. "The Therapeutics of Puberty." *AJO* 12 (October 1879).

Lyman, Eliza B. *The Coming Woman, or the Royal Road to Perfection: A Series of Lectures.* Lansing, Mich.: W. S. George, 1880.

McClanahan, A. C. "An Investigation into the Effects of Masturbation." *New York Medical Journal* 66 (1897).

McFadden, Bernarr A. *The Virile Powers of Superb Manhood; How Developed, How Lost, How Regained.* New York: Physical Culture, 1900.

Marston, L. M. *Essentials of Modern Healing.* 2d ed. Boston: The Author, 1887.

Marvin, Frederic R. *The Philosophy of Spiritualism and the Pathology and Treatment of Mediomania. Two Lectures.* New York: A. K. Butts, 1874.

Maudsley, Henry. *Body and Mind.* New York: D. Appleton, 1875.

———. *Body and Will: Metaphysical, Physiological and Pathological Aspects.* New York: D. Appleton, 1884.

———. *Responsibility in Mental Disease.* New York: D. Appleton, 1874.

Medical and Surgical Reporter 59 (September 188): 342.

Mitchell, S. Weir. *Doctor and Patient.* Philadelphia: J. B. Lippincott, 1888.

———. *Fat and Blood: An Essay on the Treatment of Certain Forms of Neurasthenia and Hysteria.* Philadelphia: J. B. Lippincott, 1877.

———. *Lectures on Diseases of the Nervous System, Especially in Women.* Philadelphia: H. C. Lea, 1881.

———. *Wear and Tear, or Hints for the Overworked.* Philadelphia: J. B. Lippincott, 1871.

Morais, Nina. "A Reply to Miss Hardaker on the Woman Question." *PSM* 21 (May 1882): 70–78.

Mortimer-Granville, J. *Youth: Its Care and Culture.* New York: M. L. Holbrook, 1882.

Napheys, George H. *The Physical Life of Women.* Philadelphia: G. Maclean, 1870.

———. *The Transmission of Life: Counsels on the Nature and Hygiene of the Masculine Function.* 14th ed. Philadelphia: H. C. Watts, 1877.

Nebinger, Andrew. *Criminal Abortion: Its Extent and Prevention.* Philadelphia: Collins, 1870.

O'Reilly, John Boyle. *Ethics of Boxing and Manly Sport.* Boston: Ticknor, 1888.

Oswald, Felix I. *Physical Education; or The Health Laws of Nature.* New York: D. Appleton, 1882.

———. "Instinct as a Guide to Good Health." *PSM* 28 (February 1886).

———. "Physical Education." *PSM* 18 (January 1881).

Pancoast, S. *Boyhood's Perils and Manhood's Curse: A Handbook for the Father, Mother, Son, and Daughter.* Philadelphia: Keystone Publishing, 1873.

Pierce, R. V. *The People's Common-Sense Medical Adviser.* 21st ed. Buffalo: World's Dispensary Printing Office and Bindery, 1889.

Posse, Nils. *The Swedish System of Educational Gymnastics.* Boston: Lee and Shepard, 1890.

Pratt, Martha L. *The New Calisthenics: A Manual of Health and Beauty.* Boston: Educational Publishing, 1889.

"The Prevention of Conception: From the Proceedings of the Detroit Medical Association." *Cincinnati Medical News* 19 (1890): 303–8.

Proctor, Richard A. *Strength, How to Get Strong and How to Keep Strong.* London: Longmans, Green, 1889.

———. "Growth and Decay of Mind." *PSM* 4 (January 1874).

Review of C. A. Green's *Build Well: Plain Truths Relating to the Obligations of Marriage.* In *PSM* 44 (February 1894): 557.

Richards, Eugene L. "College Athletics." *PSM* 24 (March 1884).

———. "The Influence of Exercise upon Health." *PSM* 29 (July 1886).

Richardson, B. W. *The Diseases of Modern Life.* New York: Appleton, 1876.

———. "Induced Diseases from the Influence of the Passions." *PSM* 8 (November 1875): 60–65.

Riggs, C. Eugene. "An Outline in the Progress in the Care and Handling of the Insane." *JNMD* 20 (September 1893): 620–28.

Sahler, Charles O. *Psychic Life and Laws, or the Operations and Phenomena of the Spiritual Element in Men.* New York: Fowler and Wells, 1901.

Saur, Prudence B. *Maternity: A Book for Every Wife and Mother.* Chicago: L. P. Miller, 1891.

Simms, Joseph. "Human Brain Weights." *PSM* 31 (July 1887): 355–59.

Sizer, Nelson. *40 Years of Phrenology.* New York: Fowler and Wells, 1891.

Skene, Alex J. C. "The Relation of the Ovaries to the Brain and Nervous System." *AJO* 14 (January 1881): 54–77.

Smith, Stephen. *Doctor in Medicine: And Other Papers on Professional Subjects.* New York: W. W. Wood, 1872.

Spencer, Edward. "The Philosophy of Good Health." *Scribner's Monthly* 4 (October 1871).

Spitzka, Edward C. *Insanity: Its Classification, Diagnosis and Treatment. A Manual for Students and Practitioners of Medicine.* New York: Bermingham, 1883.

Starr, M. Allen. "The Old and the New Phrenology." *PSM* 35 (October 1889).

Stebbins, Genevieve. *Society Gymnastics and Voice-Culture Adapted from the Delsarte System.* 6th ed. New York: E. S. Werner, 1888.

Steele, Joel D. *Hygienic Physiology.* New York: A. S. Barnes, 1884.

Stevenson, William A. "Physiological Significance of Vital Force." *PSM* 24 (April 1884).

Stockham, Alice B. *Tokology: A Book for Every Woman.* Chicago: Sanitary, 1885.

Storer, Horatio Robinson. *Insanity in Women.* Boston: Lee and Shepard, 1871.

———. *Is It I? A Book for Every Man.* Boston: Lee and Shepard, 1868.

Sully, James. *The Human Mind.* 2 vols. New York: D. Appleton, 1893.

———. *Outlines of Psychology.* New York: Appleton, 1883.

———. *The Teacher's Handbook of Psychology.* New York: D. Appleton, 1897.

Thomas, Julia, and Thomas, Annie. *Psycho-Physical Culture.* New York: E. S. Werner, 1892.

Thompson, Henry. "The Present Aspect of Medical Education." *PSM* 28 (September 1886).

Trall, Russell T. *Digestion and Dyspepsia.* New York: S. R. Wells, 1873.

———. *The Health and Diseases of Women.* Battle Creek, Mich.: Office of the Health Reformer, 1873.

———. *The Household Manual.* Battle Creek, Mich.: Office of the Health Reformer, 1875.

———. *The Hygienic System.* Battle Creek, Mich.: Office of the Health Reformer, 1872.

———. *The Mother's Hygienic Handbook.* New York: S. R. Wells, 1874.

———. *Sexual Physiology: A Scientific and Popular Exposition of the Fundamental Propositions in Sociology.* 13th ed. New York: S. R. Wells, 1872.

The Truth About Love. New York: Wesley, 1872.

Van de Worker, Ely. "The Genesis of Women." *PSM* 5 (June 1874).

Welch, William H. "Considerations Concerning Some External Sources of Infection in Their Bearing on Preventive Medicine." *Science* 14 (August 1889).

White, Frances E. "Muscle and Mind." *PSM* 35 (July 1889).

Wilder, Burt G. *What Young People Should Know: The Reproductive Organs in Man and the Lower Animals.* Boston: Estes and Lauriat, 1875.

Wilson, George. *How to Live, or Health and Healthy Homes.* Philadelphia: P. Blakiston, 1882.

Wood, Horatio C. *Brain-Work and Over-Work.* Philadelphia: P. Blakiston, 1880.

Woolson, Abba Gould. *Women in American Society.* Boston: Roberts, 1873.

Worcester, Alfred. "Gymnastics." *PSM* 23 (May 1883).

Workman, William. "The Progress of Medical Science." *Medical Communications of the Massachusetts Medical Society* 8 (1854): 291–96.

Youmans, E. L. "Editor's Table: The Relation of Body and Mind." *PSM* 4 (November 1873).

———. "Sketch of Joseph LeConte." *PSM* 12 (January 1878): 358–61.

Books and Articles by Twentieth-Century Analysts

Anderson, Perry. "The Antimonies of Antonio Gramsci." *New Left Review* 100 (November 1976): 5–78.

Banner, Lois W. *Elizabeth Cady Stanton, A Radical for Woman's Rights.* Boston: Little, Brown, 1980.

Bannister, Robert C. *Social Darwinism: Science and Myth in American Social Thought.* Philadelphia: Temple University Press, 1979.

Barker-Benfield, G. J. *The Horrors of the Half-Known Life: Male Attitudes Toward Women and Sexuality in Nineteenth-Century America.* New York: Harper and Row, 1976.

Bates, Thomas R. "Gramsci and the Theory of Hegemony." *Journal of the History of Ideas* 36 (April 1975): 351–66.

Bercovitch, Sacvan. *The American Jeremiad.* Madison: University of Wisconsin Press, 1979.

Berger, Peter L., and Luckmann, Thomas. *The Social Construction of Reality.* Garden City, N.Y.: Doubleday, 1966.

Blake, John B. "Health Reform." In *The Rise of Adventism, Religion and Society in Mid-Nineteenth Century America.* Edited by Edwin S. Gaustad. New York: Harper and Row, 1974, pp. 30–49.

Bledstein, Burton J. *The Culture of Professionalism: The Middle Class and the Development of Higher Education in America.* New York: W. W. Norton, 1976.

Bliss, Michael. "Pure Books on Avoided Subjects: Pre-Freudian Sexual Ideas in Canada." *Historical Papers.* Canadian Historical Association (1970), pp. 89–108.

Bonner, Thomas N. *The Kansas Doctor: A Century of Pioneering.* Lawrence, Kans.: University of Kansas Press, 1959.

Boyer, Paul. *Urban Masses and Moral Order in America, 1820–1920.* Cambridge, Mass.: Harvard University Press, 1978.

Brieger, Gert H., ed. *Medical America in the Nineteenth Century, Readings from the Literature.* Baltimore: Johns Hopkins University Press, 1972.

Brooks, Carol Flora. "The Early History of the Anti-Contraceptive Laws in Massachusetts." *American Quarterly* 18 (Spring 1966): 3–23.

Bullough, Vern L., and Voght, Martha. "Homosexuality and Its Confusion with the 'Secret Sin' in Pre-Freudian America." *JHM* 28 (April 1973): 143–55.

Cammett, John M. *Antonio Gramsci and the Origins of Italian Communism.* Stanford: Stanford University Press, 1967.

Carlson, Eric T., and Dain, Norman. "The Meaning of Moral Insanity." *BHM* 36 (March 1962): 130–40.

Cominos, Peter. "Late Victorian Respectability and the Social System." *International Review of Social History* 8 (1963): 19–48; 216–50.

Cott, Nancy F. "Passionlessness: An Interpretation of Victorian Sexual Ideology, 1790–1850." *Signs* 4 (Winter 1978): 219–30.

Cunningham, Raymond J. "From Holiness to Healing: The Faith Cure in America." *Church History* 43 (December 1974): 499–513.

Dain, Norman. *Concepts of Insanity in the United States, 1789–1865.* New Brunswick, N.J.: Rutgers University Press, 1964.

Davies, John D. *Phrenology: Fad and Science.* New Haven: Yale University Press, 1955.

Degler, Carl. *At Odds, Women and the Family from the Revolution to the Present.* New York: Oxford University Press, 1980.

———. "What Ought to Be and What Was: Women's Sexuality in the Nineteenth Century." *American Historical Review* 79 (December 1974): 1467–90.

Douglas, Ann. *The Feminization of American Culture.* New York: Alfred Knopf, 1977.

Douglas, Mary. *Natural Symbols.* New York: Vintage, 1970.

———. *Purity and Danger: An Analysis of the Concepts of Pollution and Taboo.* New York: Praeger, 1966.

Duffy, John. *A History of Public Health in New York City.* 2 vols. New York: Russell Sage, 1968, 1974.

———. "Mental Strain and 'Over-Pressure' in the Schools: A Nineteenth Century Viewpoint." *JHM* (January 1963): 63–79.

Earnest, Ernest. *S. Weir Mitchell, Novelist and Physician.* Philadelphia: University of Pennsylvania Press, 1950.

Englehardt, H. Tristam, Jr. "John Hughlings Jackson and the Mind-Body Relation." *BHM* 49 (Summer 1975): 137–49.

185

Erikson, Erik H. *Childhood and Society.* 2d ed. New York: W. W. Norton, 1973.

————. "The Problem of Ego-Identity: Identity and the Life Cycle." *Psychological Issues* 1 (New York 1959): 101–64.

————. "Wholeness and Totality." In *Totalitarianism.* Edited by Carl J. Friedrich. Cambridge, Mass.: Harvard University Press, 1953, pp. 156–71.

————. *Young Man Luther: A Study in Psychoanalysis and History.* New York: W. W. Norton, 1962.

Fellman, Anita Clair. "The Fearsome Necessity: Nineteenth-Century British and American Strike Novels." Ph.D. diss. Northwestern University, 1969.

Fellman, Anita Clair, and Fellman, Michael. "Man Amuck: G. J. Barker-Benfield's *The Horrors of the Half-Known Life."* In *Reviews in American History* 4 (December 1976): 558–64.

Fellman, Michael. *The Unbounded Frame: Freedom and Community in Nineteenth-Century American Utopianism.* Westport, Conn.: Greenwood Press, 1973.

————. "Approaching Popular Ideology in Nineteenth-Century America." *Historical Reflections* 6 (Winter 1979): 321–33.

————. "Rehearsal for the Civil War: Antislavery and Proslavery at the Fighting Point in Kansas, 1854–1856." In *Antislavery Reconsidered: New Perspectives on the Abolitionists.* Edited by Lewis Perry and Michael Fellman. Baton Rouge: Louisiana State University Press, 1979, pp. 287–307.

————. "Sexual Longing in Richard Henry Dana, Jr.'s American Victorian Diary." *Canadian Review of American Studies* 3 (Fall 1972): 96–105.

Fife, Austin, Fife, Alta, and Glassie, Harvey M., eds. *Forms Upon the Frontier: Folklife and Folk Arts in the United States.* Monographic Series, 16. Logan, Utah: Utah State University Press, 1969.

Fiori, Guiseppe. *Antonio Gramsci: Life of a Revolutionary.* New York: Schocken, 1975.

Foner, Eric. *Free Soil, Free Labor, Free Men: The Ideology of the Republican Party Before the Civil War.* New York: Oxford University Press, 1970.

Foucault, Michel. *The History of Sexuality: Volume I, An Introduction.* New York: Pantheon, 1978.

Freedman, Stephen. "The Baseball Fad in Chicago, 1865–1870: An Exploration of the Role of Sport in the Nineteenth-Century City." *Journal of Sport History* 5 (Summer 1978).

Freud, Sigmund. *Civilization and Its Discontents.* New York: W. W. Norton, 1962.

————. "On the Universal Tendency to Debasement in the Sphere of Love." *Standard Edition.* London, 1957, 11:177–90.

Friedman, Lawrence J. *Inventors of the Promised Land.* New York: Alfred Knopf, 1975.

Fullinwider, S. P. "Insanity as the Loss of Self: The Moral Insanity Controversy Revisited." *BHM* 49 (Spring 1975): 93.

Geertz, Clifford. "Ideology as a Cultural System." In *Ideology and Discontent.* Edited by David E. Apter. New York: Basic Books, 1973.

Genovese, Elizabeth Fox, and Genovese, Eugene D. "The Political Crisis of Social History: A Marxian Perspective." *JSH* 10 (Winter 1976): 205–20.

Genovese, Eugene D. *In Red and Black.* London: Penguin Press, 1971.

Gilbert, Arthur N. "Doctor, Patient and Onanist Diseases in the Nineteenth Century." *JHM* 30 (1975): 217–34.

Gilbert, James B. *Work Without Salvation: America's Intellectuals and Industrial Alienation, 1880–1910.* Baltimore: Johns Hopkins University Press, 1977.

Goffman, Erving. *The Presentation of Self in Everyday Life.* Garden City, N.Y.: Doubleday, 1959.

Gordon, Linda. *Woman's Body, Woman's Right: A Social History of Birth Control in America.* New York: Grossman, 1976.

Gordon, Michael, ed. *The American Family in Social Historical Perspective.* 2d ed. New York: St. Martin's, 1978.

Gottschalk, Stephen. *The Emergence of Christian Science in American Religious Life.* Berkeley: University of California Press, 1973.

Greven, Philip. *The Protestant Temperament: Patterns of Child-Bearing, Religious Experience and the Self in Early America.* New York: Alfred Knopf, 1977.

Grob, Gerald N. *The State and the Mentally Ill: A History of the Worcester State Hospital in Massachusetts.* Chapel Hill, N.C.: University of North Carolina Press, 1966.

————. "Mental Illness, Indigency and Welfare: The Mental Hospital in Nineteenth-Century America." In *Anonymous Americans: Explorations in Nineteenth-Century Social History.* Edited by Tamara K. Hareven. Englewood Cliffs, N.J.: Prentice-Hall, 1971, pp. 250–79.

Hale, Nathan, G., Jr. *Freud and the Americans: The Beginnings of Psychoanalysis in the United States, 1876–1917.* New York: Oxford University Press, 1971.

Haley, Bruce. *The Healthy Body and Victorian Culture.* Cambridge, Mass.: Harvard University Press, 1978.

Haller, John S., Jr. "Neurasthenia: Medical Profession and Urban 'Blahs.' " *New York State Journal of Medicine* 70 (October 1970): 2489–93.

Haller, John S., Jr. and Robin M. *The Physician and Sexuality in Victorian America.* Urbana, Ill.: University of Illinois Press, 1974.

Harper, John Paull. "Be Fruitful and Multiply: Origins of Legal Restrictions on Planned Parenthood in Nineteenth-Century America." In *Women of America: A History.* Edited by Carol Berkin and Mary Beth Norton. Boston: Houghton Mifflin, 1979, pp. 245–69.

Hartman, Mary, and Banner, Lois, eds. *Clio's Consciousness Raised: New Perspectives on the History of Women.* New York: Harper and Row, 1974.

Himes, Norman E. *Medical History of Contraception.* New York: Schocken, 1970.

Hoare, Quentin, and Smith, Geoffrey Nowell, eds. *Selections from the Prison Notebooks of Antonio Gramsci.* New York: International, 1971.

Hollinger, David P. "Historians and the Discourse of Intellectuals." In *New Directions in American Intellectual History.* Edited by John Higham and Paul Conkin. Baltimore: Johns Hopkins University Press, 1979.

Horowitz, Daniel. "Consumption and Its Discontents: Simon N. Patten, Thorstein Veblen, and George Gunton." *Journal of American History* 67 (September 1980): 301–17.

Jackson, Stanley W. "Force and Kindred Notions in Eighteenth Century Neurophysiology and Medical Psychology." *BHM* 44 (September and November 1970): 397–410; 539–54.

Judt, Tony. "A Clown in Regal Purple: Social History and the Historians." *History Workshop* 7 (Spring 1979): 66–94.

Katz, Michael. *The Irony of Early School Reform: Educational Innovation in Mid-Nineteenth Century Massachusetts.* Cambridge, Mass.: Harvard University Press, 1968.

Kaufman, Martin. *Homeopathy in America: The Rise and Fall of a Medical Heresy.* Baltimore: Johns Hopkins University Press, 1971.

Kelly, Robert. *The Cultural Pattern in American Politics: The First Century.* New York: Alfred Knopf, 1979.

Kemble, Howard R. *The Great American Water Cure Craze, A History of Hydropathy in the United States.* Trenton, N.J.: Past Times Press, 1967.

Kennedy, David M. *Birth Control in America: The Career of Margaret Sanger.* New Haven: Yale University Press, 1970.

Kett, Joseph. *The Formation of the American Medical Profession, The Role of Institutions, 1780–1860.* New Haven: Yale University Press, 1968.

Kraditor, Aileen S. "American Historians on Their Radical Heritage." *Past and Present* 56 (August 1972): 136–53.

Leavitt, Judith Walzer, and Numbers, Ronald L., eds. *Sickness and Health in America: Readings in the History of Medicine and Public Health.* Madison: University of Wisconsin Press, 1978.

Marcus, Stephen. *The Other Victorians: A Study of Sexuality and Pornography in Mid-Nineteenth-Century England.* New York: Basic Books, 1966.

May, Elaine Tyler. *Great Expectations: Marriage and Divorce in Post-Victorian America.* Chicago: University of Chicago Press, 1980.

Meyer, Donald B. *The Positive Thinkers: A Study of the American Quest for Health, Wealth and Personal Power from Mary Baker Eddy to Norman Vincent Peale.* Garden City, N.Y.: Doubleday, 1965.

Mohr, James C. *Abortion in America: The Origins and Evolution of National Policy, 1800–1900.* New York: Oxford University Press, 1978.

Morantz, Regina Markell. "Making Women Modern: Middle Class Women and Health Reform in Nineteenth-Century America." *JSH* 10 (Summer 1977): 490–507.

Morgan, H. Wayne, ed. *Yesterday's Addicts, American Society and Drug Abuse, 1865–1920.* Norman, Okla.: University of Oklahoma Press, 1974.

Neuman, R. P. "Masturbation, Madness and the Modern Concepts of Childhood and Adolescence." *JSH* 8 (Spring 1975): 1–27.

Nissenbaum, Stephen W. "Careful Love: Sylvester Graham and the Emergence of Victorian Sexual Theory in America." Ph.D. diss. University of Wisconsin, 1968.

Numbers, Ronald L. *Prophetess of Health: A Study of Ellen G. White.* New York: Harper and Row, 1976.

Papanek, Hanna. "Purdah: Separate Worlds and Symbolic Shelter." *Comparative Studies in Society and History* 15 (June 1973): 289–325.

Park, Roberta J. " 'Embodied Selves': The Rise and Development of Concern for Physical Education, Active Games and Recreation for Women." *Journal of Sport History* 5 (Summer 1978).

Parker, Gail Thain. *Mind Cure in New England: From the Civil War to World*

189

War One. Hanover, N.H.: University Press of New England, 1973.

Pellegrino, E. D. "Medicine, History and the Idea of Man." *Medicine and Society. The Annals of the American Academy of Political and Social Sciences* 346 (March 1963): 9–20.

Penfield, Wilder. *The Mystery of the Mind.* Princeton: Princeton University Press, 1975.

Perry, Lewis. " 'Progress, Not Pleasure, is Our Aim': The Sexual Advice of an Antebellum Radical [Henry C. Wright], *JSH* 12 (Spring 1979): 354–66.

Pivar, David J. *Purity Crusade: Sexual Morality and Social Control, 1868–1900.* Westport, Conn.: Greenwood Press, 1974.

Rather, L. J. *Mind and Body in Eighteenth Century Medicine.* Berkeley: University of California Press, 1965.

Reed, James C. *Private Vice to Public Virtue, Birth Control in America, 1830 to the Present.* New York: Basic Books, 1978.

Rein, David M. *S. Weir Mitchell as a Psychiatric Novelist.* New York: International Universities Press, 1952.

Reverby, Susan, and Rosner, David, eds. *Health Care in America: Essays in Social History.* Philadelphia: Temple University Press, 1979.

Risse, Guenter B. et al., eds. *Medicine Without Doctors: Home Health Care in American History.* New York: Neale Watson, 1977.

Robinson, Paul. *The Modernization of Sex.* New York: Harper and Row, 1976.

Rodgers, Daniel T. *The Work Ethic in Industrial America.* Chicago: University of Chicago Press, 1978.

Rosen, George. *A History of Public Health.* New York: M. D. Publications, 1958.

Rosenberg, Charles. *No Other Gods: On Science and American Social Thought.* Baltimore: Johns Hopkins University Press, 1976.

———. *The Trial of the Assassin Guiteau: Psychiatry and Law in the Gilded Age.* Chicago: University of Chicago Press, 1963.

———. "And Heal the Sick: The Hospital and the Patient in Nineteenth-Century America." *JSH* 10 (June 1977): 428–47.

Rosenkrantz, Barbara G. "Cart Before Horse: Theory, Practice and Professional Image in American Public Health, 1870–1920." *JHM* 29 (January 1974): 55–73.

Rossi, Alice, ed. *The Feminist Papers.* New York: Bantam Books, 1974.

Rostow, Walt Whitman. *The Stages of Economic Growth: A Non-Communist Manifesto.* London: Cambridge University Press, 1960.

Rothman, David J. *The Discovery of the Asylum: Social Order and Disorder in the New Republic.* Boston: Little, Brown, 1971.

Rothstein, Abraham. *American Physicians in the Nineteenth Century.* Baltimore: Johns Hopkins University Press, 1972.

Ruddick, Sara, and Daniels, Pamela, eds. *Working It Out: 23 Women Writers, Artists, Scientists, and Scholars Talk About Their Lives and Work.* New York: Pantheon, 1977.

Ryan, Mary P. "The Power of Women's Networks: A Case Study of Female Moral Reform in Antebellum America." *Feminist Studies* 5 (Spring 1979): 66–85.

Schrank, Robert. *Ten Thousand Working Days.* Cambridge, Mass: M.I.T. Press, 1978.

Scott, Donald M. *From Office to Profession: The New England Ministry, 1750–1850.* Philadelphia: University of Pennsylvania Press, 1978.

Sears, Hal D. *The Sex Radicals: Free Love in High Victorian America.* Lawrence, Kans.: Regents Press, 1977.

Shryock, Richard. *Medicine in America: Historical Essays.* Baltimore: Johns Hopkins University Press, 1966.

Sicherman, Barbara. "The Uses of a Diagnosis: Doctors, Patients, and Neurasthenia," *JHM* 32 (January 1977): 33–54.

Sklar, Kathryn Kish. *Catharine Beecher: A Study in American Domesticity.* New Haven: Yale University Press, 1973.

Smith-Rosenberg, Carroll. "The Hysterical Woman, Sex Roles and Role Conflict in Nineteenth-Century America." *Social Research* 39 (Winter 1972): 652–78.

———. "Sex as Symbol in Victorian Purity: An Ethnohistorical Analysis of Jacksonian America." *American Journal of Sociology* 84 Supplement (1978): S212–47.

Stanton, William. *The Leopard's Spots: Scientific Attitudes Toward Race in America, 1815–1859.* Chicago: University of Chicago Press, 1960.

Takaki, Ronald T. *Iron Cages: Race and Culture in Nineteenth-Century America.* New York: Alfred Knopf, 1979.

Thomas, Lewis. "A Meliorist View of Disease and Dying." *Journal of Medicine and Philosophy* 1 (1976): 212–21.

———. "Notes of a Biology Watcher: The Health-Care System." *New England Journal of Medicine* 293 (December 1975).

Turner, Victor. *The Forest of Symbols.* Ithaca, N.Y.: Cornell University Press, 1967.

Walsh, Mary Roth. "The Quirls of a Woman's Brain." In *Women Look at Biology Looking at Women.* Edited by Ruth Hubbard et al. Cambridge, Mass.: Schenkman, 1979, pp. 103–25.

191

Walters, Ronald G. *American Reformers, 1815–1860*. New York: Hill and Wang, 1978.

———. *Primers for Prudery: Sexual Advice to Victorian America*. Englewood Cliffs, N.J.: Prentice-Hall, 1974.

Warner, John Harley. "The Nature Trusting Heresy: American Physicians and the Concept of the Healing Power of Nature in the 1850s and 1860s." *Perspectives in American History* 11 (1977–78): 291–324.

Whorton, James C. "Christian Physiology: William Alcott's Prescription for the Millennium." *BHM* 49 (Winter 1975): 466–81.

———. "The Hygiene of the Wheel: An Episode in Victorian Sanitary Science." *BHM* 52 (Spring 1978).

Wiebe, Robert H. *The Search for Order, 1877–1920*. New York: Hill and Wang, 1967.

Williams, Gwyn A. "The Concept of 'Egemonia' in the Thought of Antonio Gramsci: Some Notes on Interpretation." *Journal of the History of Ideas* 21 (October 1960): 586–99.

Wollheim, Richard. *Freud*. London: Fontana, 1971.

Wright, Gwendolyn. *Moralism and the Model Home: Domestic Architecture and Cultural Conflict in Chicago, 1873–1913*. Chicago: University of Chicago Press, 1980.

Young, James Harvey. *The Toadstool Millionaires: A Social History of Patent Medicines in America Before Federal Regulation*. Princeton, N.J.: Princeton University Press, 1961.

Young, Robert M. *Mind, Brain and Adaptation in the Nineteenth Century: Cerebral Localization from Gall to Ferrier*. Oxford: Oxford University Press, 1970.

Index